Fibromyalgia

Journeys

A Collection

Stories of Courage

and Personal Triumph

Compiled by Shelly Bolton

New Dawn Publishers, 2013

Printed in the United States of America

Contents

Prologue

Do you know what it is to deal with fibromyalgia...really? This disorder that touches every corner of the lives of those living with it can be incredibly difficult to describe. Sometimes the best way to describe such a concept is through examples-glimpses into the lives of those who know it first-hand.

Here we have assembled a collection of true stories from a sampling of people affected by fibro. These accounts come from a wide variety of people of different ages and from very different walks of life. Each is affected by this disorder in a different way and to a different extent, and each has different coping strategies.

The main thing these folks have in common is that they are each bravely facing a daily life of pain and challenge, and they do not let it beat them! Each fighter represented here is achieving their own victories by living their lives around their challenges. Each person's triumphs are different, ranging from getting to the bathroom without assistance, to working outside the home, to walking a marathon. At each level of ability, however, overcoming whatever obstacles exist must be seen as a victory!

Each story or poem is told from the unique perspective of the individual, and hopefully each one will give you a new viewpoint from which to understand the journey of anyone who is living with this disorder.

Superwoman

By Laura Gage

Most days I wake up and think of myself as Superwoman. On Monday, I woke up 20 minutes late, because I apparently hit my snooze button 3 times without even remembering it, but no sweat...I mean I did at least finally wake up! I sit up in my bed and realize that my covers are all in a twist, and my neck and back are covered in sweat. No wonder I feel so tired! I must've had a rough night.

I put my feet on the floor, and as they take on the weight of my body, I realize that they really hurt!! I'm not worried though, this is my norm, and I know that this foot pain of mine goes away after a while as I move around getting myself ready for the day. I go to the bathroom first thing, because my bladder is about to explode. I rinse my mouth out with water from the bathroom faucet, because -just like every morning- it is so dry I can't even swallow. I walk slowly into the kitchen, laughing at myself for moving like an 80 year old when I am only 39. I sit at the kitchen table and flex my fingers and hands for 5-10 minutes. They are so stiff and swollen I can't use them yet, and I need to make my coffee.

After I feel I have enough movement and strength in my hands I make my way over to the coffee maker, noticing that my feet are still hurting. I make my coffee, but apparently too soon because I spill coffee grounds all over the counter and floor when the scoop drops from my poor hands. Crap, guess I should've exercised them a little longer, but by this point I am in a hurry. I already overslept, and even though I showered last night I know I will need a bath before I go into work... first, because I woke up covered in sweat, gross; second, my feet are still hurting and my hands are still stiff, so I know a tub soak is what I need before I can move forward with my day.

I finally am dressed, and I'm off to work. First though, I need to get a glass of water for the drive. I only work ten minutes away, but I never go anywhere without something to drink because I have the worst dry mouth on the planet. I drive to work in silence, because when I listen to the radio on the way it sometimes gives me a headache, and I don't want to chance it. As I drive I notice that my lower back is really achy, and I've got those weird sharp pains shooting through my calves again.

I get to work, ten minutes late, no makeup, hair in a ponytail. I feel like Superwoman! I made it. I can do anything. Against all odds, I continue to amaze myself! I fancy myself a martyr. People just don't know what someone like me has to go through just to get to work every morning!! They take such small things for granted, but I am a champion, because no matter how bad I feel I am still working and taking care of my family every day!! Then I encounter other people, and I get the looks. Those looks that tell me I am late again and it's annoying. Those looks that say "Can't she at least put on make-up and fix her hair before she comes to work?" The giver of the looks that day could be anyone; it may be co-workers, could be the boss, might be a customer, who knows? Sometimes it might even be my husband or one of my children.

I feel my throat tighten a little, but swallow it down. I tell myself I'm probably just being overly sensitive today because I don't feel well. A remark: "You don't look well today." The questions: "Are you feeling bad again?" "Your fibromyalgia bothering you today?" Sounds harmless on paper, I know. It's not the questions or the remarks that are hurtful, it's the tone. Gone are the sympathetic eyes, gone are the reassuring smiles. The questions and statements are laced with exasperation. The most fatal is when a child or loved one asks, "Are you feeling good today?" ...not with a tone of hopefulness, not because they think you might be, but in a tone that is desperate and begging. The question becomes a plea. I hear "PLEASE FEEL GOOD TODAY!" And I do want to, I really, really want to! So I lie, and I swallow my pain and fatigue, and I smile and say, "I'm fine, why?" In that moment, I feel like Superwoman.

It is not my personal unhappiness, but the unhappiness of those whom I love -and who love me- that bothers me. I want to scream, and cry, and shout at the top of my lungs " I CAN'T HELP IT!! MAYBE I LOOK LIKE CRAP, MAYBE I'M LATE, BUT I MADE IT! I GOT OUT OF BED TODAY, I GOT DRESSED, I MADE COFFEE, AND I DROVE HERE!! I MADE IT THROUGH THE DAY IN 15 MINUTE INCREMENTS, TALKING MYSELF THROUGH IT!! STOP LOOKING AT ME LIKE I AM WEAK AND PITIFUL!! I AM STRONG!!! I DO THIS EVERY DAY!!!" I listen while people I love, respect, and admire tell me stories about this person who has Fibro and doesn't take any medications. This other person who has Fibro and exercises all of the time, and this one person who knows a lot of people who have fibro, but they just push through the pain. "This one article I read said it's your diet." "Are you taking vitamins?" "Are you sure you have Fibro?" "Maybe you're just depressed." "You should change your diet." "You should really start exercising." All the while, I'm smiling, and nodding, and agreeing. All the while, I'm shouting in my head, "DON'T YOU KNOW? CAN'T YOU SEE I'M SUPERWOMAN? DON'T YOU KNOW I AM PUSHING THROUGH THE PAIN? DON'T YOU KNOW I HAVE READ ARTICLE AFTER ARTICLE? DON'T YOU KNOW I GOT A SECOND OPINION, EVEN THOUGH I DON'T HAVE INSURANCE, AND I COULDN'T REALLY AFFORD IT? DON'T YOU KNOW I SUFFERED WITH THIS FOR 5 DAMN YEARS BEFORE I EVER EVEN WENT TO THE DOCTOR, OR TOOK ANY MEDICINE? Don't you know that it took me 2 years after being diagnosed with this to even talk to anyone outside of my family about it, because I was confused, and ashamed? Don't you know that before the Fibro, when you all thought I was Superwoman, I really wasn't...that part was easy? Don't you even realize that I am Superwoman NOW?"

By days end, or weeks end my illusions of grandiosity are over. Sure I made it through the week, but I was late twice and left early twice. Sure, I'm working every day, but not as a Nurse, as I was trained to do. Sure, I keep getting up and going through the motions, but I can't keep my house clean or my laundry caught up. At the end of the week, I'm a failure. My whole self-identity, self-worth, self-esteem has forever and always been wrapped up around being a strong, smart, independent woman who gets things done, because they have to be done.

This disease, syndrome, illness, whatever it even is, has changed all of that. I do not even know how to be this person that I am now. I haven't even had a chance to ask myself how I feel about it. I wake up on Monday morning, and I feel like Superwoman. By Saturday, I feel like a huge failure. Somewhere in between, I muster up the strength to do it all over again.

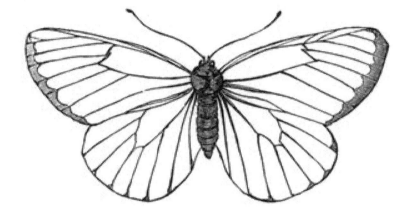

Land of Confusion

By Connie Papp

Where to begin? First of all, I was only recently diagnosed with fibromyalgia, in the summer of 2013. I was told prior to that I have Polymyalgia Rheumatica and some symptoms of Fibromyalgia, but had not received an official diagnosis. I have experienced chronic widespread muscle pain, brain fog and extreme fatigue since February 2012. I began having muscle spasms, pain that moves around my body, occasional tremors and disorientation while driving in August 2012.

I will begin by mentioning strange symptoms leading up to the onset of my chronic pain, because I feel they were the precursors to the onset of the disease. Approximately 2 years ago, I began having strange "cattle-prod-like" jolting pains across the tops of my feet. The jolting was so intense at times, my feet would actually jerk and twitch. This continued for approximately a year. At or around the same time period, I noticed it was becoming more and more difficult to sit for long periods of time. I needed to lean on my desk, or arm of a chair, or armrest in a car to assist in rising to a standing position. The pain and stiffness were intense, but after walking awhile the pain would ease a little. In contradiction, when I would walk too long, my hips would groan miserably! I thought at

*the time, "Wow, really?...I'm only 52!" I come from a long line
of very strong women; so of course, I pushed on and just dealt
with it. I eventually went to my PCP, had x-rays and was
diagnosed with "possible left sided sacroiliac arthritis." It
didn't seem like much to worry about at the time since the
diagnosis contained the word "possible."*

*I don't really have time for anything beyond typical pain. I am
a Community Manager for 9 homeowners associations. That
may not sound like much, but if you are a member of a HOA,
I'm the "bad guy." I have to be the bad guy and manage every
facet of an HOA, which is a corporation, and all the
responsibilities that entails. I don't just have one boss or a
couple of bosses. I answer to approximately 1,600
homeowners, 9 Boards of Directors, and manage all their
requests, calls, emails, demands, pay all their bills, manage
their finances, coordinate insurance claims and deal with
astoundingly rude, inconsiderate, angry, threatening, cursing
people! I also attend board meetings after my work day is
done, several nights a month, which equates to a 12+ hour
day. In addition, I chair annual meetings, budget ratification
meetings and assessment increase meetings. These are only a
FEW of my responsibilities. My job is a giant stress ball and I
jokingly tell people, "I juggle ferrets." Managing my job is an
ongoing struggle all while having constant pain, blinding fog
and heavy exhaustion, however I'm still working.*

I have had my share of emotional turmoil after not one but two marriages to alcoholics / addicts. I believe there was something broken inside me... I didn't love "me" enough and wasn't emotionally or spiritually healthy enough to choose a healthy person. After going to Al-Anon for 5 years and realizing I didn't have the power to change anyone but myself, I still tried. That... is the definition of insanity. I believe the suffering I endured attempting to help both alcoholics / addicts, took a devastating toll on my health. If you've lived with an addict you are familiar with the depth of emotional turmoil I'm referring to. Emotional suffering must manifest physically. I believe this with every fiber of my being. To add insult to injury, I am also a "sensitive" and am very sensitive to other people's energies, good and bad. I literally feel what other people feel, intensely, as if the feelings were my own.

If I haven't bored you to death and you're still with me, let me share what I refer to as, "the beginning of the end." In February of 2012, I had just returned home from Miami after spending some time with my fiancé, who was in training for a new job. I just remember feeling horribly sick and out of sorts, but I kept pushing on as usual. Every muscle ached, I felt feverish, I couldn't think clearly, and I was experiencing an all-encompassing exhaustion like I'd never felt before. The intensity of these symptoms went on for 2 weeks. The brain fog is probably what frightened me the most. I remember driving to a meeting on February 15, 2012, because the meeting was noted on my work calendar. When I arrived at my meeting, I didn't remember how I got there. I was trying to wrap my head around what was happening to me, but it was beyond any illness I'd ever experienced.

Besides the symptoms I mentioned I experienced a couple of years prior and a hysterectomy at the age of 33, I had always been a healthy individual. I studied classical ballet and been an instructor for 20 years of my life. I was a "go-er and do-er!!" I had boundless energy! I pushed through everything and kept rolling! What the heck was wrong with me? I looked at my best friend one day and couldn't find the words to describe how horrible I felt and how completely freaked out I was. Instead, I began to cry. No... I sobbed. These were gut wrenching tears and feelings that come from the depths of your soul. The pain and fear engulfed me. When I managed to stop crying, I whispered, "I don't know what's wrong, but something is very, very wrong with me... and I'm afraid." I didn't dare say it out loud because I instinctively knew, deep inside, this was no typical illness.

I decided at that point to make an appointment with my PCP. I dragged myself to his office, cried and recited all my symptoms. I stated I felt very strongly it was not the flu and implored him to help me. He listened calmly to my plight and sent me to the lab. He prescribed 25 mg of Prednisone per day for five days and told me to return in two weeks. If anyone reading this has ever taken Prednisone, you know it cures anything that ails you! I began feeling much better during this five day treatment. However, once the Prednisone was gone all the symptoms returned. I scheduled another appointment with my PCP before two weeks had passed.

At this point, my suspicions were confirmed. I knew this was not the flu or anything like the flu. My PCP was evidently concerned as well, because it was written all over his face. He suggested I research Polymyalgia Rheumatica, prescribed more Prednisone and referred me to a rheumatologist. It took two months to get the appointment. I still had pain, fog and exhaustion even taking the Prednisone. The pain was less intense, but the fog and exhaustion seemed unaffected.

I was treated by the rheumatologist for almost a year with very little help. My experience with the first rheumatologist was disappointing, but I've learned that I have to be my own advocate and I will not waste any more precious time with a Dr. that does not prove he's actively involved in helping me achieve at least a better quality of life. My rheumatologist referred me to a Neurologist for the disorientation while driving. The results of a neurocognitive test have showed that I have short term memory loss and slow reaction time.

I have recently been referred to a new rheumatologist and he at least has expressed concern and has a plan of action.

As I sit here pondering all that has transpired in the last 16 months I realize I have been through a lot. It feels like I'm reading about someone else's life…..but it is my own. My poor body has worked so very hard to support me and I am so very grateful. I am also grateful I have support from my loved ones. I realize not everyone has support that is so desperately needed. For that, I am very saddened. I wish support and love for all of us who suffer with chronic pain. I still have hope that one day we will no longer suffer. I still believe a cure or at least relief is possible.

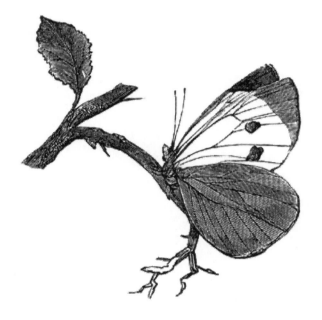

THE MONSTER IN ME

By Kelli Coleman Glover

What is this monster that lives in me? It steals so much of my life away and causes misery

It comes to me as pain and fatigue; it comes as a stomach crushing with a fit of rage

It plays on my skin like pins and needles, it grabs my head as if it were in a vice grip on a carpenters table

What is this horror story my life has come to be, of nights without sleep; but I need sleep more than I ever have, will slumber ever come?

Now I have a repeat nightmare to chase away: Will that ever go away?

What is this light so bright and smell so overwhelming? Every fiber I feel sends shocks up my skin that send me yelling

Sounds and smells, Bright lights and crowds; it is all too much to take, when your senses have no brakes

Many family and friends think I am attention seeking , if they could just be me for a day, they would know the true overwhelming pain and collateral damage this monster is wreaking

Judgment and stigma would be removed, if they only knew what it is really like

To sit up in the long hours of the black of the night; alone and in pain but not a noise I can make

The time I spend curled in a ball with a hot pack as my best friend

My partner in life who shares this hell and carries the weight of life's responsibilities and demands

This monster dictates my life and I should not have to prove it, but alas! I do, I have this horrible condition and I hope it never finds you!

What is this rasp upon my voice? What are these aches in my fingers and toes? What is this ache? Down my arms they go! Oh No! The dreaded flare!

Now the pain is amplified and the senses multiplied; the pain is horrifying to the point you want to die. No hope left in your soul and you have nowhere to go.

As if the monster wasn't enough, it flares its ugly head and gets worse

It feels as if you are walking with heavy balls chained to your legs, it feels as if you have been beaten to a pulp

Will this monster ever ease, will the stigma ever stop? Will there be awareness and compassion and a cure, I pray! I hope and pray that someday, someday... this horrible monster will go far, far away

For inside me is a girl with a colorful, bohemian twirl

I want to frolic in fields of flowers and dance in the sun

I want to hike up great mountains and chase the sun into the night

I want to play in the ocean, running in the tide

If my body could do what my soul is feeling, I would be unstoppable

Unshakable

A firecracker

No one could keep up with me

But the monster wins each battle, each and every time

It is a force I cannot reckon with so I hope in time,

There is cure, a treatment... something to help

Because I have a lot of living left to do, the monster may win the battle, but it will not win the war!

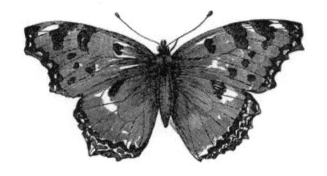

Keep Walking

By Brandi Dukes

My name is Brandi, and I am a 30 year old woman living in the eastern Midwest.

I was always healthy as a child- never sick; no broken bones. I had some back pain issues since the age of twelve, just due to how I was built. I had some issues like headaches and sometimes got dizzy, and I was sensitive to extreme temperatures. There were a lot of tests in my teen years to see what was causing the headaches and dizziness, but when no cause was found it was labeled migraines and I just had to learn to live with it- but I was otherwise healthy.

Everything changed my freshman year in college. I had some anxiety issues that started at eighteen, and during my freshman year I was assaulted- causing my anxiety level to skyrocket. I dropped out of school and withdrew from life for a while, living like a hermit and putting on weight. When I did start getting back out there, I began living a very destructive lifestyle. I started drinking a LOT and then at 20 I got pregnant. I had a traumatic delivery which left me in the hospital for almost a month. After that I never seemed to get back to the way I was prior to the pregnancy. The scattered and foggy "pregnancy brain" seemed to morph into what I now know as "fibro brain."

The physical pain began gradually, and when I talked to doctors about it the only response I ever got was that I should lose weight. I maxed out at 200+ pounds and, out of discouragement, quit seeking out medical help and just suffered in silence. The anxiety kept getting worse, to the point that I once had to leave my daughter's birthday party because it got so bad. I've left carts full of groceries trying to escape it. I finally was able to lose weight- and lost over 70 pounds, hoping the doctors had been right and that it would fix everything. It didn't- the pain and anxiety were still there, and were actually getting worse.

Having lost weight I was finally able to find a doctor that would listen to me and help find answers. He did a lot of blood work, a sleep study, and countless other tests. He was at first hoping that if he could get the sleep problems fixed then that would take care of the rest. Since I was young and healthy, he figured the lack of sleep had to be the cause of all, or at least most, of the other problems. After about a year of doctor visits and tests, we finally had a diagnosis. I had developed so many symptoms, and little did I know that they would all end up fitting precisely into the description of fibromyalgia. In fact if you looked at a list of my symptoms, it is exactly the list you would find if you googled "fibromyalgia symptoms."

Sleep is still my biggest issue, and that leads to constant and debilitating fatigue. Even when I can at times get extra sleep, it seems no amount helps. I fight sleep all day and have to get up and move frequently just to avoid falling asleep at my desk, and there is no time of the day that it is better or that I feel more "high energy." I get up and walk in the mornings, and walk more at lunch. Then sometimes I walk again during my daughter's gymnastics practice- but nothing ever seems to help.

As for treatments, my doctor is still trying to find the right combination of medications to help, and he has referred me to a pain specialist as well. When we first started out we tried Paxil to help with the anxiety, which it did- but I promptly put on twenty five pounds. You know, those pounds I worked so hard to get rid of? Yep, those pounds! I'm currently on Cymbalta for the hip pain but the help is minimal. Flexeril helps me sleep, but I still never feel refreshed. I take a multivitamin (One A Day) which actually does seem to help with the brain fog- it doesn't get rid of the memory problems, but at least I feel more mentally clear. I'm also on Gabapentin, which helps keep symptoms to a manageable level, which I suppose is all I can ask for. No cure. Just getting by. I would love, just occasionally, to feel rested and awake.

How this has affected my personal life:

I used to be very outgoing and I loved doing things with my family and friends. Now... I try not to commit to anything because I never know what I will be able to follow through with. I am both a mom and a wife, and my family tries their best to understand, although I constantly feel as though I'm letting them down. We simply cannot do as much as we used to, and I am always so tired that my husband takes over most of the home responsibilities.

I have friends as well, who go back and forth between being concerned about me and being frustrated. I don't do anything with them in the winter because it is just too painful. They all got together right before Christmas to take the kids sledding and I had to stay home because there was just no way I could endure it. They tried to talk me into it, saying there was a fire pit, not understanding that the cold goes all of the way to the bone. It's not like I can just put on an extra layer of clothes. It even hinders my ability to walk. I feel like I disappoint people a lot, and I hate constantly feeling that I'm letting someone down.

Thankfully I am able to work full time. As bad as I feel all of the time I just cannot imagine not being able to work. If I were home all the time with nothing to do but feel sorry for myself, I can say with certainty I would spiral downward and it would be bad. I am someone who needs the mental distraction of work. I have had physical jobs before, cleaning office buildings after hours, and I would be in pain and in tears a lot of that time. Now I work at a desk job and sit at a computer- and if anything I hurt more. I have to get up about once an hour and move around, do stretches at my desk, and some days just sit in front of the computer and cry.

For a while I coped by drinking alcohol- and with my medications that is not a good combo! I have left the alcohol behind now. I do spend a lot of time in bed, and I spend more time than I would like watching television, which I find embarrassing. I do try to work out when I can- and I am trying, in the warmer weather, to get ready for a 5 K for this summer. The warmer weather helps but some days it is just physically impossible to train, so though I hope to finish the whole thing, I don't really have the full expectation of it.

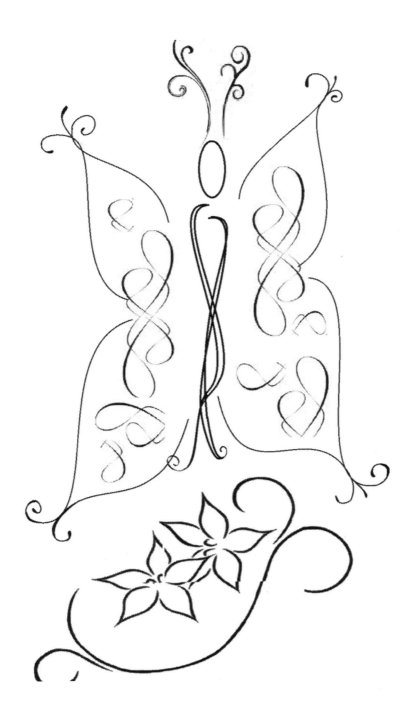

A Curse and a Blessing

Cassie Behrendt

Since fibromyalgia awareness is something this world needs to take more of an interest in, I wanted to explain what living with chronic pain is like, and what better way to do that than to tell my story? So here is my curse and my blessing...

Chronic pain is unlike anything I have ever experienced in my life. It's nothing like pain from a surgery or from an injury. It's relentless. There is no light at the end of the tunnel, no physical therapy, medication or time can heal my pain. It is with you every moment... every second... of everyday.

It took me, a problem-solving, hardworking overachiever, and it broke me. Years later and I am still trying to put the pieces of my life back together. My dreams became unachievable, my life forever difficult, forever changed.

People stepped out of my life; they didn't understand. Having lived it myself I realize they couldn't possibly!

How do you explain to a healthy person what my life is like each day? That I awake each day to a nightmare? Each morning my 27 year old body feels like an 80-year-old's. Waking up feels like I have been run over by a Mac truck several times. Getting up sounds like rocks shifting into place... Snap, crackle and pop.

Your body feels weighted down by hundreds of extra pounds when you're struggling to get out of bed. Exhaustion sets in and showers turn to baths. It's not just constant unrelenting pain and fatigue that you live with either. You experience constant headaches and migraines. You battle bladder, stomach and nausea problems on a daily basis, and the bathroom has become your friend and third most visited place in the house besides the couch and your bed. You're out of breath and struggle to walk small distances or climb stairs. You experience brain fog, have memory problems and have lost intelligence. At times being able to think or concentrate becomes an impossible task.

You can never experience comfort again and can find no comfortable place, position or clothing. Doctors and hospitals become all too familiar. There are always medications, blood work, lab work, and testing. Medical bills are always coming. Older and wiser family members ask you what they can expect from ultrasounds, cystoscopies, colonoscopies, laparoscopies, MRIs, etc... Depression sets in because even simple, daily tasks become too difficult and too much to bear. Restless legs keep you up at night. Sleep can be unreachable or you can't get enough. The bed has become a restless place filled with tossing and turning all night long.

You will never get a break from your reality because no vacation is a getaway from your daily battle, your worries never left behind. Each day the whole world continues to go on around you when you feel as yours has ended. You spend each day watching everyone around you live a life you can no longer dream of. This is my curse.

But as each day goes on it becomes a bit more bearable; you stop looking back on the life you once lived and begin to look towards the future. You find your joy in the simple things in life. You come out of the fog you were once living in and open your eyes to the incredible beauty of the world around you.

You see what others do not. You have more understanding and a profound compassion. You begin to not judge others, not knowing what secret life may be going on behind closed doors. You try and smile more and be grateful for everything in your life you do have. You truly appreciate and love those who stood by your side; they are now your true friends, your true family.

Through turmoil and strife you have finally become the person you have always wanted to be. This is my blessing.

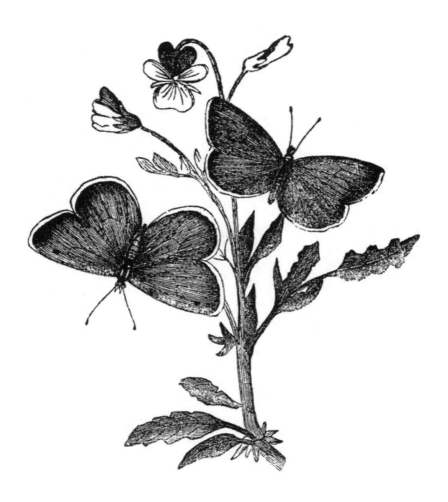

Never Give Up

By Dawn Santos

In my early 20's I became increasingly more fatigued than I had previously been. My concentration was off. My muscles were sore all the time. I did not sleep well, and felt as though my life was always moving too fast and it took all my energy to keep up with it. I was trying to juggle a small child, college classes on and off, parties with friends on the weekend, and I worked- sometimes multiple jobs. So when I looked for a reason why I felt the way I did, it was obvious. The stress of being a young single parent and all the responsibilities that come with it was always number one on the list. Working at a health club, babysitting weekend nights and staying up all night were all next in line. I went to counseling to learn how to manage my life and although it was somewhat helpful, I was told I had Adult ADD , that I was bi-polar, and had manic depressive tendencies. After trial and error with multiple medications and lifestyle changes nothing ever really improved. So I gave up.

In my early 30's when my second child was a year old I came down with meningitis. After this episode I never seemed to fully recover. Widespread body pain and fatigue were ruling my life. Most days I was forcing myself to stay on my feet and get through the day, get chores done, and not look weak or lazy. I was now married and had more responsibility and could not figure out why life seemed so unfulfilling. Yet another year later the signs of meningitis reared their ugly heads and I was back at the hospital for a second time. By now I think I am a medical mystery, an anomaly. I began to do less and less of things I enjoyed, became anxious in certain situations, and withdrew from friends. I suffered from injuries and winter illnesses that seemed to never want to heal or go away. I finally decided something was wrong with me and it must have been the meningitis.

I searched the internet, read books from the library, and although I realized I do in fact have ADD, there were too many other possibilities out there for me to diagnose myself with anything. Finally I decided I didn't know what was wrong with me but I knew changing my diet would be nothing but helpful. I did that and no change really made much of a difference. In between numerous doctors' appointments with dismissive answers, my in home daycare children, foster children and my own third baby, I ended up having to scale back and eventually quit everything to just sit home and be sick. I felt like a failure and a loser. I felt weak and ashamed that my body could not keep up with everything my heart wanted to do. In seeing a Rheumatologist for another injury, he quickly changed his line of questioning, did the tender point test and diagnosed me with Fibromyalgia. I went home searched the internet to find out exactly what that was and then had my greatest "aha" moment in 5 years. I was happy to have diagnosis that validated me. I was not crazy! Then I cried. It seemed I was doomed to a life of pain with no cure in sight. The emotional fallout was much greater and more complicated than I can ever put into words. I ended up on disability and just plain miserable.

At 39 I decided to try diet change again but his time I would be more strict. No artificial ingredients, no caffeine, GMO (genetically modified foods), HFS (high fat/sucrose), etc., and as few processed foods as possible- as clean as I could afford. This time it made a noticeable difference. Right away I felt like I had a little more energy, and I was less heavy, angry and also had fewer digestive issues. I felt good enough to start running and working out again, as I had done in the past, but then it became too painful. Shortly after that, when bringing my youngest to preschool I met another mom there who was a doctor. We got a little friendly and after a few of my side handed comments like "I'm always so tired," and "everything hurts," she said she would love to see me (as a patient) and try to figure out what was going on. I declined for a while. Besides the fact that it had the potential to be awkward, I was suffering from doctor fatigue. I did not want to go through that anguish of hearing "its tendinitis, I have to lose weight, it *will go away eventually, or all new moms feel like this". Then I figured what do I have to lose?*

She did testing no one had ever done before. I had Fibromyalgia for sure, but also some overlapping Chronic Fatigue Syndrome. I had Hypothyroidism, and had Adrenal Fatigue. Other side conditions from the high stress and wacky hormones also developed, like TMJ and anxiety. Throughout this process I discovered it all led back to the birth of my first child. I had been living with this for an astonishing 22 years; all the while it was getting worse with every stress or trauma. She put me on supplements specific to my needs based on those tests and a thyroid medication. I exercised a minimum of 30 minutes a day, 5 days a week. It hurt. It was not easy. But every day I could do a little more and a little more. Sometimes I cried while I ran around the track, other times I yelled at the TV and cursed the maker of the DVD, but it was helping me. I could see it and feel it. And combined with the healthy diet I felt like a human again.

I decided to be in control. If I could not cure it I would mold it. I was in pain anyway, so I decided I would benefit from it by building a stronger body for it to live in. Feeling sore from a workout is mentally and emotionally more empowering than feeling the pain from Fibro itself. Although there are "flares" and bad days sometimes, life is much better. I have less pain and less depression. I was able to start working and start a support group. I started an organization for people with who suffer with chronic pain who also stay active. They get together for events, give support, suggestions and share stories of accomplishments. I never would have been able to get any of this done without educating myself, having the support of a good doctor and a supportive family.

My advice to anyone is to know you are you are important. Your life matters. No one will fight for you as hard as you will fight for yourself so do not give up. Keep looking for the right doctor, vitamins, or exercise. Try everything alternative as well as modern. Know it will most likely be a combination of things that help, just as it is a combination of things that are making you ill. It may take months or years but it's worth it. You have to form a front on every level- physical, emotional, mental and spiritual so it has no chance but to back down. I know it hurts. Don't give up.

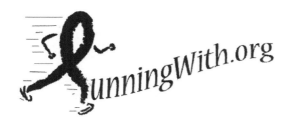

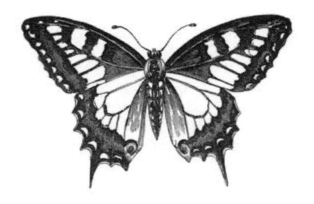

The Chronic Pain Poem

By Lara Greco (Yume)

Seven AM – I lie awake,

Here's my medicine to take,

Should I pop it, should I skip it,

Should I man up and just endure it?

Eight o'clock, the alarm rings,

I gotta do a lot of things,

There's the laundry, a list of chores,

Prep the kids, and mop the floors.

Nine AM, I take more meds,

Just too sore – I made the beds!

So let me sit and rest a bit,

I am much more tired than I admit.

Ten o'clock,

I phone the doc,

"Can I have one more refill?

Yes, next month I'll pay the bill."

At eleven I get up,

Let me try to walk the pup.

Right, my physio said it's good,

But my legs just feel like wood.

Midday comes, it's time for lunch,

I could use some thing to munch.

But cutting stuff is out of the question,

So I eat crackers and depression.

1 PM, I take more pills,

Side effects give me the chills.

I lay again, just for a second,

Or, at least, that's what I reckon.

I wake once more at 3 PM,

Kids come home, I stay with them.

I try my best to look quite happy,

While instead I feel just crappy.

Make them a snack, then dinner's baking,

Cooking hurts, my hands are aching.

Other half comes back from job,

Sense of guilt could make me sob.

Pop more drugs right after food,

But these ones affect my mood.

I'd like to sleep and just forget,

But the day's not over yet.

I gotta plan tomorrow's stuff,

Maybe three pills will be enough?

I need to drive and buy some things,

If pain just doesn't kill my limbs.

When I get to bed, I'm tired and sore,

I say a prayer, and hurt some more.

At four AM again awake,

A cramp that makes my body shake.

If you think this can't be true,

Then I'm sorry, you have no clue!

Might there be sun, might there be rain,

This is life with CHRONIC PAIN.

(www.survivingchronicpain.com)

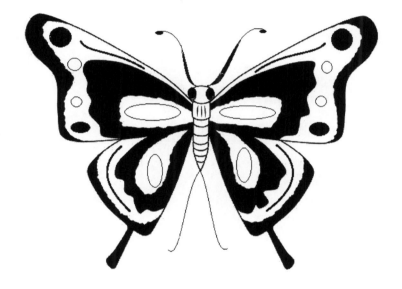

Youth is Not Exemption

By Natalie Frew

My name is Natalie and I am a 20 year old student living in New Zealand. I am working on my bachelor's degree for Science (Technology) with a double major in Biological Sciences and Biochemistry. This all goes to my life's goal, which is to be accepted to medical school so I can become a doctor and help others.

Though I was quite accident prone and had severe 'growing pains' as a child, I was otherwise fairly healthy. I also had glandular fever at fifteen which damaged my immune system, so I do get sick fairly easily since then. My mum is a nurse and my dad is an orchard manager. My dad had prostate cancer when I was twelve, for which he was treated in another city, and thankfully went into remission the following year. He now has rheumatoid arthritis due to the hormones he was treated with. I also have a sister who has ankylosing spondylitis, and both she and dad have swelling around their joints, which is not something I have experienced. We do however have in common some stiffness and my sister and I both have some issues with spinal range of motion.

At 17 I began to have cramping and shooting pain in my right knee when I crouched. As there was no injury or trauma I knew this was not normal. The pain then spread throughout the rest of my joints and muscles. I also have some brain fog with word confusion, major fatigue, abdominal cramps and insomnia. Otherwise I find that I do not have some of the same issues as other fibromyalgia patients, though I do experience depression and anxiety. I have seen approximately seven GPs and three rheumatologists, and was originally diagnosed with non-specific arthralgia. The fibromyalgia diagnosis came two years after my first doctor appointment for these issues, just before my nineteenth birthday. The spinal range of motion issues are just now being investigated so I am currently awaiting a rheumatologist appointment for this.

I struggle with attending all of my classes, and I do the majority of my studies from home. I find myself limited in the usual social activities of college students, and even just getting around on campus. It takes a mental and emotional toll as I am trying to study full time and get high grades that will allow me to be accepted to med school, and I often feel that I am being judged because of my limitations; I feel that people just think I am lazy since they don't understand how debilitating this condition is. I do work full time since I am required to complete 1200 hours of placement employment as part of my degree, but I find that I do not have enough energy for anything else. Since I cannot be on my feet for long or do much lifting or other heavy physical tasks, I must work at my own pace and not try to necessarily keep up with the pace of other workers.

I have a boyfriend of seven months and have explained my condition to him, but since he lives in another town he is not really around enough to fully understand the effects on my life. My sister and father are fairly understanding since they both struggle with physical issues, but my mum is not quite so understanding. She regularly tells me that I am being a drama queen or that it is all in my head, though I am sure she doesn't intend to be hurtful. Thankfully my best friend -and flat mate- understands and really watches out for me, making sure that I eat and don't push myself to hard, and she helps me when I am having a difficult day.

As far as treatments, I have tried amitriptyline, which I could not continue because it sedated me too heavily and I could not function. I have also tried nortriptyline, SSRI antidepressants, other antidepressants, NSAIDS and other pain meds, as well as others, none of which were helpful. The only treatment which has helped is Tramadol, but the relief from it is minimal. I have begun going to the gym three times per week and have had a workout designed for me based on my specific issues, and I hope to see some physical benefits.

I like to watch TV, listen to music, and spend time with friends. I also enjoy using social media networks like Tumblr. I have joined a few Facebook support groups and have connected with some other fibro sufferers my own age there and on Tumblr. I find this helpful, since most people with fibro are in their thirties and forties, and they struggle with different things than me and others my age.

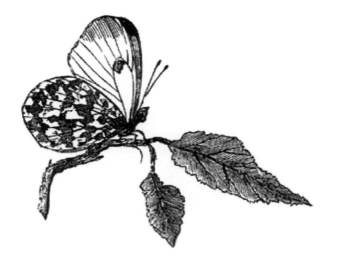

Stepping Stones to a Different Path

By Kelli Coleman Glover

My name is Kelli Coleman Glover and I am just a few weeks shy of turning fifty years old. I have never dreaded decade birthdays, but for some reason I am really dreading this one. Perhaps it is because I thought my life would go down a completely different path than it has led. Perhaps it is because I feel my life is so meaningless since I have become fully disabled. I feel like I am more of a burden than I am worth. I think most of all it is because I feel closer to ninety years old most days than fifty. Fibromyalgia will do that to a person. It is a cruel, mean condition. As I look back, I can see what I would call little stepping stones that led to my final diagnosis at age thirty two and then a precipitous turn about fifteen years later that had me completely disabled. Did these stepping stones contribute to my fibro-filled life? Did these stepping stones cause my life to become one that is dictated by my illness? It is my theory that my illness is like a line of dominoes which fell one by one until I arrived: life dictated by fibromyalgia.

I grew up in Bakersfield, California, a (then) medium size city about two hours north of Los Angeles. The first ten years of my childhood could only be described as what I would call my "Wonder Years". Bakersfield is known for being hot. In fact in

Bakersfield, we invented hot! Summer days are generally over 100 degrees Fahrenheit. I loved it nonetheless. I lived in the blue collar part of town and we played all day, bare footed.... riding bikes, playing hide-and-go-seek, chasing the ice cream man and playing in the sprinklers until dusk when our moms would start hollering our names out one by one to come home. I had wonderful family. They made even the smallest things fun! Do not get me wrong, I had some very dark things happen to me in my early childhood, but if I could lift those dark things out, it would have been a pretty 'as good as it gets' childhood.

As a child my health was generally good. I got an occasional cold as anyone does. The only thing I really had trouble with was my tonsils. Every year I had at least three bouts of tonsillitis. About the age of ten things started to change in many areas. I went through a very accelerated growth spurt and started getting frequent migraine headaches. These migraines would continue and never let up. In fact in the last few years, they have precipitated to the point I get a headache everyday .... and at least 5-8 migraines a month. I also had terrible and unbearable growing pains in my legs. The closest thing I can compare it to would be: it was like I had a migraine in my calves. My dad would sit at night in the hot house as the breeze of our swamp cooler wafted slowly over me and just rub and rub my legs. My dad was a great man and one of the most influential and important people to ever grace my existence. Easter break of 5th grade (also age ten), I finally got those pesky tonsils out. The surgery went well and my throat infections were reduced to almost non-existent.

When I was ten one of the biggest negative influences in my life also started; my mom started drinking wine on a daily basis. It became heavy drinking and within months she was a full blown functioning alcoholic. I hated it! I despised everything about it.... the smell, the sound of the cork opening, the sound of the wine glass hitting the table, the slur in her voice but most of all the way it made her act. She turned mean. By the time it got to this point I was in the sixth grade and eleven years old. She decided to use me as her 'best friend' and confide in me things no eleven year old... especially a daughter... should ever hear. Her drinking was and still is one of the biggest obstacles to my emotional healing I face, even today. This was also the start of my extreme anxiety and bouts of serious depression. And if that were not enough, when I was thirteen, we sold the little, comforting house 'that built me', moved from the blue collar part of town to the posh part of town (my mom wanted prestige!) and my parents divorced. My world was spinning out of control. I was a chubby, awkward girl with no money and suddenly no friends in a school full of preppy rich kids... that were strangers to me. The dominoes were beginning to fall.

As my High School years began, my days grew darker. My parents' divorce shattered my world. My mom began dating a man that I did not like very much. He was not mean but he was just bland. He had no personality at all. My father and my two uncles (one of whom I was very close to) were lively, fun, zany and just made everything lighthearted. This man was like a dry cracker. My mom ended up marrying this man and with that I did acquire a step brother who was one year older than me and a step sister who was one year younger than me. We got along for the most part... although my step sister was quite into the 'uppity' lifestyle and made no bones about it. I was and always will be much closer to my step brother who is a great, down to earth guy.

My mom's drinking continued throughout my high school years and it weighed on me as if I were carrying an elephant on my back. I found refuge in chorus and drama and was mortified every time we had a concert or play because she would show up sauced. Why couldn't she just wait two hours! Just two hours for that stinking vino! I was embarrassed and wanted to run away and hide. She was loud and brash. So it would make sense that I had my first panic attack during one of my choral concerts. Being tall, I was always on the highest rafter. It was awful! I thought I was going to pass out. I became frightened beyond words. I felt like the walls were closing in yet I was so high off the ground I was going to come tumbling down and pass out. I felt as if I could not breathe and my chest was caving in. I thought I was going to die! Somehow I managed to make it through and from that moment on I would have panic attacks without a moment's notice anywhere, anytime for any reason. My anxiety was out of control and I am sure the emotional turmoil of my mom's drinking was a large part of why this was happening. Anxiety and all, I wanted to continue my path on the stage and become a professional opera singer. I did have the voice for it but would have had to proceed like all professionals; train, practice and work at it for hours on end each and every day. I took private lessons, entered vocal solo festivals. I tried out for every play and solo part. Also, I managed to lose about thirty pounds and maintain a healthy, normal weight my last two years of High School. I started dating with wild abandon and got engaged on my eighteenth birthday to a young man I had been dating for six weeks. I really did love him as much as any eighteen year old can love in that capacity. We got married in January of 1982. I was eighteen years old and he was twenty years old. He was an apprentice pipe fitter and I, just out of High School, had a job as a bank teller. So with that went both my college education and my dream of singing. I do not blame him. Part of me was in love with the idea of love, babies and 'doing it right!' and part of me just had to get out of that house of horrors. Even if I had proceeded to college (I was accepted and was going to start going to the University in my hometown), I would have continued to date this young man. So at the time, I saw my future with him. My goal was to marry, get out of my mom's house and then go to college part time at night. Money was tight, but we managed to make ends meet. I still struggled with panic attacks... never going to the doctor for them. I never had even heard of them at this point. I thought there was something unique with me that no one else had and I did not want to be locked up, so I suffered in silence. I would continue with night school and end up with over fifty college units, but it is obvious, I did not get my degree and I certainly did not become a famous singer. Meanwhile, I started putting on weight. My weight would dominate most of my adult life and in fact I would be considered obese for the better part of my adult life. In March of 1983, I had a miscarriage at about ten weeks into my first pregnancy. I wanted a baby to love so very badly. I was devastated beyond words. It took me a year to get pregnant again but God blessed us with a baby two weeks before Christmas... our little Christmas miracle. She was perfect. We had three more girls in the next eight years and though we did not plan it that way, of course I would not change a thing.

In September 1988 when my second daughter turned two years old, I had a terrible bout of bronchitis. About a month after this, I was diagnosed with costochondritis: an inflammation of the rib cage which can cause severe chest pain. The doctor suspected my bronchitis had been the culprit. Could this have been one of my stepping stones? Could this have been a domino falling? This condition is a common thread of fibro patients, but it would be seven years before I would be officially diagnosed. Something happened during my last pregnancy that I believe is crucial in my journey with fibromyalgia. When I was eighteen weeks pregnant (at age 29), I got the chicken pox. Now one might laugh at this, nevertheless, approximately one hundred people a year die from the chicken pox (caused by the varicella zoster virus). Also given the fact that I was eighteen weeks pregnant, I was so scared my unborn daughter might be harmed. Four weeks later at twenty two weeks pregnant, it got even worse..... I got the shingles! I have been studying fibromyalgia for a long time and have talked with many people who have fibromyalgia. There is one statement nearly 100% of all fibro patients can complete: "I was never the same after _____." For me, I was never the same after having the chicken pox and shingles as a pregnant adult. This is where I feel my true walk, as I know it, with fibromyalgia began.

Let the dominoes start falling. When my youngest daughter was two months old we had just moved into our first (bought) home. Imagine having four feisty, bright and spirited girls aged eight and under... three of them in sports and two of them in school. Imagine your husband suddenly decides he wants a dog, right then, right now. Imagine there are boxes and more boxes and everything is 'in a box.... somewhere'. I was diagnosed with depression and put on Prozac. I would remain on it for the next seven years, still hailing it as one of the best things I ever did! So I have the depression thing under control and the boxes are pretty well unpacked and about six months later I noticed my hips were tender. I usually noticed this during my daughter's feedings. This was not painful at the time, just strange. Following that, my neck started hurting. This pain was bad. I had never felt pain this bad in the day to day sense except for my migraines. I went to my family doctor who took x-rays of my neck and I remember exactly what he said, "You are having severe muscle spasms. The spasms are pulling on the neck and causing a reverse curve. We need to send you to a Neurologist." We of course now know that a reverse curve is called kyphosis. I will touch more on that later.

When I saw the Neurologist (in Bakersfield), this began my long, frustrating walk with doctors and how difficult it is to find a doctor that knows how to treat fibromyalgia and/or even thinks it is a real disorder. The doctor I saw initially told me he thought I had a condition that mostly affected 'middle aged' women. At this time, I was only thirty one years old and considered fairly young to have this 'disorder' he called fibrositis (remember, this is 1996). He decided to send me down to Scripps Institute in La Jolla, CA. It was at this time however, something else was in the works. We were considering a move... across country. So in between seeing the initial doctor (in Bakersfield) and going to Scripps we flew out to Roanoke, VA so my husband could see what this job offer was all about. We also could see the area and decide if we wanted to leave our lifelong home and move to the other side of the country. It was a beautiful place and lovely to visit but as I have since learned along the way, always listen to your gut. My gut screamed at me, "Don't move! Don't move". Gut scream or not, the offer was accepted and the kids and I would join my husband in June. After we got home from our visit to Virginia, within a few weeks we went to Scripps in search of a diagnosis about why my neck and shoulders were in such agonizing pain. One of the neurologists at Scripps confirmed Fibrositis/Fibromyalgia, after a very long, grueling and extensive exam.

So I have this thing I cannot even pronounce... I remember them writing it on a piece of paper for me, as I sat numb. Now what do I do? All this! And faced with three months of having to be a 'single' parent and prepare for a cross country move. I broke down into tears. It probably seemed a little over the top for the doctor, but in the context of my world it was just all too much, too fast. First, he gave me a cocktail of medications; a low dose prescription pain pill, a muscle relaxant and a high dose of anti-inflammatory medication (800 mg. Ibuprofen). Second, he gave me a series of exercises. Third, he recommended counseling to help with my anxiety and depression. It was like I was outside myself watching someone else. How could I remember all of this? Was this really happening? What is a chronic condition anyway? Will it go away? Will it get worse? I had a million questions in my head, but like Ralphie trying to ask Santa for that Red Ryder BB gun, I suddenly became tongue tied and unable to speak. For someone who rarely shuts up, I could not utter a word. I just sat there and shook my head like a dazed animal. Over the years I would see numerous doctors on every end of the spectrum. I would see good, bad, and utterly clueless. For the most part I would be lucky... mostly because I would not let myself settle for anything less than what I or any human being deserves, good and respectful health care. What a long, strange and sometimes frustrating trip I was about to embark on with this new... fibromyalgia. I know most every person with fibro can relate to this, the only difference is I would come to have twenty years of relating under my belt.

A few months later we made the big move. Now moving is stressful enough. However, moving with four little girls ages two years old to eleven years old is overwhelming. Each has to be registered in school. We had to find a new pediatrician. We had to find a new church. We had to find the grocery store. We had to find our way around town. Most of all, I had to find a new doctor. God blessed me there and I got it on the first hit! My first doctor here was actually a man who had fibromyalgia himself! While I hated to see anyone else go through this hell, this doctor was very understanding. Things went along well. My protocol was going good. I still had pain but the cocktail I was on seemed to be keeping the pain levels manageable. Most days I was maybe at a level four (oh, how I long for those days now). About a year after we moved, I started having what would forever be known as my 'stress knot'. My stress knot is on the right hand side of my neck and when it spasms, it hurts, burns and pulls so badly, I want to cry out in pain. It is also in such a bad state that it can both be felt and seen. It looks like a small walnut under the skin. This would be the introduction of my trigger point injections that I would continue to get over the

66

years. It is my understanding these shots have a steroid and lidocaine (a numbing agent) in them and serve to break up the spasm. They worked beautifully! So when they would get to that point, I went in for these injections and probably averaged two to three a year. It was also after the move that my fatigue levels began to rise and the doctor added Chronic Fatigue Syndrome to my diagnosis... explaining to me that many doctors consider fibro and CFS one in the same condition. At this time I was sleeping several hours during the day after sleeping eight to nine hours at night. I sometimes slept up to fourteen hours a day. This is when my marriage really started hitting a bad patch and started its downward cycle.

I know without doubt my husband's family thought I was exaggerating if not making up my illness. My husband defended me (at this time) to some extent. This was my first introduction to the stigma surrounding fibro. As my marriage began to suffer more and more, I began to plead with my husband for marriage counseling. During this time we were informed that the factory that moved us to Virginia would be closing and sending us to South Carolina, about six hours south of Roanoke. Another move! All the same, this move would mean a warmer climate. The damp weather of Virginia was starting to greatly impact me. This area would be in the deep south and nice and toasty! So once again, we moved. I found a job there, part time, that I loved. I liked it there but my husband did not so when this fickle company decided they 'made a mistake' by closing the initial plant, they gave us the option of moving (yet again!) back up to Virginia. I did not want to go, I loved my job and I loved the endless sun that only the deep south could bring. It appears I had no say. We moved back anyway. The stress of my dying marriage and constantly moving was taking its toll on my fibro.

It was within two years of this move that my marriage really went downhill. There was no hope. The next several years of my life would prove to be the most pivotal regarding where I am today; totally disabled by my fibromyalgia and how it dictates my life. There go more and more dominoes just falling and falling.

The ugliest, saddest, most hateful divorce in the history of man ensued. In the next few months I began to work in a pay day loan center. I had been a stay-at-home mom for nearly twenty years... working part time off and on... but no steady current work skills. The pay was not very good, but it was a foot in the door. Only five months later, one of the customers recruited me to come work in a large bank call center for which she worked. The pay would be $3 an hour more and I would have good benefits. For the first time in my life I would live as an independent, self-sufficient woman.

In 2005 I remarried the most kind, gentle, understanding man on earth. He is my best friend. He came into this marriage with full awareness of my fibromyalgia. He knew that it would only get worse, never better. He knew everything; the good, the bad and the ugly. Most of all, he loved me. I was a good 100+ lbs overweight and it did not matter. He loved me for who I was, not for what size dress I wore. I had been working at the call center and had good insurance so I decided to branch out and get a pain management specialist. This doctor was very good and kept me on the same basic protocol, except he gave me Topomax to help stop my numerous migraines before they started (about five to ten a month). I stayed with this doctor for many years and his treatment was adequate, though my levels on most days would be at about a six on a 'good' day and a seven or even an eight on a bad day! I went along for about three years with this doctor even trying an epidural in my neck. I decided to undertake something very life-altering... I made the decision to have Gastric Bypass. It had been my dream my entire life to lose weight and it was going to come true! After ten months of jumping through hoops the insurance required, on February 5, 2007 early on a frigid morning, I was rolled into the operating room, giving my husband a big grin and two thumbs up. It was successful! I initially lost over 150 lbs. I thought the weight loss would prompt a big turn around in my fibromyalgia. It did not. The one constant thing in this journey from hell is pain.

The year I had my gastric bypass (2007) is when things really started to go downhill. The dominoes started to fall quicker. A chain of events began to unravel and with each chain, my illness took a bigger and bigger hit. Four months after my surgery, the day after Father's Day 2007 at 2 AM, our phone rang. We were dazed as anyone would be with a 2 AM phone call. The caller ID had my cousin's name and it was coming from California. My dad had passed suddenly at the young age of sixty seven years old. He had been very ill with his diabetes but never let on to me in our many wonderful and long phone calls that there was a problem. I was crushed and to this day I sometimes wonder if I will ever get to the 'acceptance' stage of grief. My dad's death took a great toll on me and it was about this time that the neck issues really started getting worse. I was having these spasms and knots nearly every day and they were also exasperating my headaches. My husband became what I called 'my favorite medication'. He took up reflexology and started doing foot-rubs for me every single night. He also rubbed my neck and shoulders as needed. It was and still is the time of day I look forward to the most.

Shortly after my dad passed away, my job at the call center was outsourced and I went to work for another call center. Sadly, my insurance changed and my pain management doctor did not accept my new insurance. This is when things really became bad as far as doctors go. I started with a new pain management doctor whose office felt more like a 'cattle call' than a waiting room. They pushed as many patients into an hour as they could, and unless you were going to get a lecture that day you never got your fifteen minutes. This doctor did not listen to what you had to say and he was curt and smug to boot. Nonetheless, there was no choice. He kept me on the same protocol but something happened to change all that and it went from bad to worse! In 2010 I fell on black ice in the parking lot at work. I was sent to the doctor work had contracted. He gave me opiate pain medication and sent me to a specialist because my arm was in pretty bad shape. I would come to find out I had a periosteal contusion (deep bone bruise) in the upper arm and had to keep it immobilized for five weeks. I called my pain management doctor twice to let them know what was happening. My husband was standing right next me as I made both calls. I also asked the doctor my employer sent me to call the pain clinic.

My pain management doctor says he never received any of the
calls. Since I called twice and the other doctor called once, I fail
to believe he missed three calls. Even so, I had two choices, be
dismissed from the clinic for 'breaking my contract' or go
through a Suboxone treatment center. I chose the latter.

In August 2010 I began a Suboxone treatment program. I went
to all the meetings, cleared all the urine screens and saw my
counselor without fail. Though the Suboxone was keeping me
from going into withdrawal, my pain levels were starting to
spike and I was getting introduced to the wonderful world of
'fibro flares'. I was suffering from flares often and knowing I had
unfairly been put into a program I did not deserve due to poor
phone handling, I was a nervous wreck. On top of that I was still
grieving over my dad's death. All the same, I completed the
program with flying colors and was released back to the doctor
and told I could go back on opiates. He did not see it that way.
He thought Suboxone was the only way and this would remain
my treatment for the next three years. He maintained it was the
'best and strongest' pain medication available as he saw it and
that if I did not like it, I could 'go somewhere else'. Things were
really taking a bad turn. Work was so stressful. I was having
asthma attacks several times a week. I had migraines at least
five or six times a month. My IBS was keeping me from getting

out of the door almost every day and when I did get to work I would have to sign off my phone sometimes three to five times an hour. My brain fog was starting to overtake me and at times I could not think straight. My anxiety was out of control and I was working closely with both a counselor and a Psychiatrist. My commute was an hour drive each way and I was starting to get pulled over from erratic driving (because I was so consumed with fatigue). It was all too much! Then came the straw that broke the camel's back. On September 30, 2010 I was only about 10 minutes from home. This was a rare day at the call center in that it was not stressful. I was driving home down the country road when I felt the car shaking. The next thing I knew I was over-correcting; the car flipped on its roof, and then back on its wheels. I sat for a moment in a daze. I had a gash in my leg.... a pretty bad one, but other than that I was OK. I was not cited, as a tire blew causing the accident. The dominoes were really falling now and I was in the middle of it. I did not know it was going to get even worse.

A few weeks after my accident, the gash in my leg was not looking very good. Ironically it was my counselor at the Suboxone program I was going through that noticed how bad it was. She was a lovely woman and we got along beautifully. She suggested I get my leg seen to immediately. I was not prepared to hear what they were about to tell me: I had an MRSA infection in my leg. I was scared stiff! I had read about MRSA recently in the paper. Two kids at my daughter's high school had died from this thing! I was taken out of work yet again because of the severity of the wound and how serious it was to treat. I had to soak it in wet, sterile compresses three times a day for an hour at a time and dress it each time. I had giant horse pills. I had to watch it like a hawk for any sign of change. They did not take this lightly at all and with my already compromised immune system this was very critical because one wrong thing happening and things could get really bad really fast. I still, to this day, have a round 'scar' of sorts on my right leg. I call it my 'badge of honor'. I do think the MRSA infection was a pivotal turning point in taking my illness from difficult but manageable to fully disabling.

I continued through the Suboxone program and finished with flying colors. I was the only person in my group that did not either miss a class or bust at least one urine screen (which they did every meeting, three times a week). I was released to go back to Dr "Non-Understanding". My fibro was worsening at a precipitous rate and I was fully disabled out of work after exhausting my FMLA and my doctors concurred that I could not work anymore as of January of 2011. My clinic counselor wrote,

"Is ready and able to resume opiates and our recommendation at this time is that she do so". The doctor did not care. Not only did this suit with an ego not listen when I told him I did not want to be on something so strong; he would intercede, "There is nothing better for pain!" even though Suboxone is not a pain medication. When I asked for other options he would quip, "Warm Pool! You need warm pool therapy!" I explained, "That would be nice... if I could afford it." He never listened... ever.

I proceeded to have two surgeries over the couple of years between going back to him and what I would call my 'final battle' with him in which he did something so unethical that I had no choice but to seek other avenues. The first surgery was a partial hysterectomy. The second of the two surgeries found me missing my Granddaughter's first birthday because I was busy having my life saved. Ignoring the "No NSAIDS!" rule of post gastric bypass for years (due to all the headaches, thank you fibro), I perforated my intestine where it connected to the pouch (post gastric bypass). Most people do not have to be a health care professional to know: that is life-threatening serious... as in life-altering serious. On July 2, 2011 I was CAT scanned at about 3 AM. I was in an OR at 5 AM. I remember the doctor, a man I had never met, pacing up and down and he kept repeating, "This is bad, this is really bad." He was older and stuttered a bit. I have never been so scared in my life. I would come to find out he was one of the most esteemed surgeons in the area and we would grow to have a great doctor/patient relationship. I was in the ICU for three days and had what I call one of medicine's greatest torture devices, the nasal/gastric tube, for five days. Though they probably would have liked to have kept me another day or two, it was by my strong resolve that I was out of hospital in one week. It took me months to fully get back to 'my normal'. In fact I would go as far to say it was a good year before I was really back to 'my normal' and it was after this event that I never have been below a pain level seven. This event was huge in the decline of my fibromyalgia. Many, many more dominoes fell after this huge, emergency surgery.

One of the biggest and most difficult was the death of my mom, suddenly, out of nowhere. I got the call on a Monday night. My step-sister called and told me she had passed and did not know all the details. The next five days are what will forever be described as the most 'manic-numb' of my life. My mom and I had not spoken for ten years and it was not because I was trying to punish her or hurt her. No. I just could not be around the addiction. She had done many things in my life that some would call 'deal breakers' but all were forgiven. I knew she had a very tough childhood and that she was struggling with demons of her own. I asked only one thing of her: Get help for her drinking and I would be her biggest fan. She quit drinking the day she died. Just because you have not had contact with a parent does not mean their death does not hurt. In fact in many ways her death had more of a sting than my dad's passing. My dad and I were close and even though he hid his the extent of his illness from me, we were good and he left this earth knowing that. With my mom, she left this earth still choosing the wine. Her death still haunts me. Losing both my parents inside three years really took a toll.

Once I got back from burying my mom, I continued to fight to get off the Suboxone. Despite the fact that with both surgeries and various tooth abscesses I was able to go an opiate medication and go right back on the Suboxone (and I was on a strong opiate for three weeks after my abdominal surgery), 'Dr McNot-Listening' would not budge. I called my former pain doctor one day because I had a 'light bulb' moment: I now had insurance through my husband's job that my first pain management doctor accepted and I thought I could go back to him! I was crushed to learn he had retired. No! So I kept with the current doctor that I tolerated and stayed on this medication that I both felt was way over the top and did not help my pain to the extent other medications could; it was, after all, a medication made to ease withdrawal from opiates and even heroin. I would tell him every time I went for my visit that I wanted off this horrible train wreck; he never listened. This went on for just over two years and in that time I went from bad to barely able to cope on days. Finally in 2012 after months of pleading and practically begging to have this issue escalated to someone else to look for other problems above and beyond the fibro, this doctor agreed to send me to a Neurologist to have further tests run on my neck. I had been given numerous trigger point injections and three epidural procedures with only mild temporary relief from two of the epidurals. The two collective test found the following: Two fully herniated discs, degenerative disc disease, several bone spurs, stenosis on every level of the C spine down to T-1, Kyphosis (a bow or reverse curve in the neck), osteo-arthritis and so many things out of line that nerves are pinched causing numbness in my hands and feet and beginning to cause me to take unscheduled falls. Besides fibro, I now have what would be called 'tangible' issues... things that can be seen on scans and tests.

I had proof! I had documentation! Pictures do not lie, Especially two different scans- both an MRI and a CAT Scan. First, I wanted to have copies of each page gilt-edged and certified mailed to every person that accused me of making up my pain including every member of my ex-husband's family. So, more dominoes fell, and this time it was an entire stack. There was only one surgeon in our area of nearly 300,000 (with two teaching hospitals) that would agree to take the surgery. I would have to think long and hard about Anterior Cervical Discectomy and Fusion in my C-Spine. After all, my fibro would still be here and I have heard numerous negative things about this surgery. The doctor was great. I loved his bedside manner and his reputation is as good as it gets. I am not ready now and do not know when I will be. I let the surgeon know I will let him know when I am ready to have it... when that time ever comes.

That finally brings us to the most recent events and the most unethical display by a doctor I have ever witnessed. After years on Suboxone and years of endless daily headaches and muscle knots in my neck, during a recent appointment this doctor proclaimed his unhappiness; I was too frightened to make a change. By this time, fibromyalgia was front and center. From the pain of the morning stiffness to the fatigue and knotted neck of night, fibro rules my life. The one thing I learned is if your gut is screaming at you, listen and obey! This doctor did not like the way my psychiatrist was treating me and the medications he was using. Furthermore he demanded I sign a release. He started explaining how the Drug Enforcement Administration was 'requiring psychiatric records' for being able to write a prescription for Suboxone. None of it sounded right to me. I told him I did not feel comfortable signing a release that contained very personal and dark information. As I sat there crying like a baby, he was crass... cold... uncaring. He almost enjoyed it. He stated that unless I signed this release that he would not write my prescription. Blackmail? Really? He was bullying me! I was mad! Furious! I was crying so hard by now I was shaking. He wanted me off one medication that my Psychiatrist was prescribing. What business of it was his? None. I was making some great progress, albeit painful progress, it was good all the same. I was having recurring nightmares and repressed memories were coming back to me like pictures in flash shots. What my Psychiatrist prescribed to me for reasons that were needed was between him and myself and it was in no way, shape or form any business of this doctor. I finally signed... under duress. Shaking and crying as I signed. Upset does not begin to describe it. I then promptly went home and called the DEA. It was a lie. An outright lie!

My husband and I decided the best thing to do would be to see my Family doctor and tell him what happened and go from there since he had to put in a referral to another pain management doctor. He did not think there would be any problem with any pain management getting me off the Suboxone onto something else because it is not really a pain med, you have to have a special license. To top it off it is a very potent medication. While it never 'drugged me up', this medication also did not help me with my pain. It kept me from going into withdrawals but for two years I was having the worst pain of my two decades with this beast of a disorder. So the day finally arrived after mountains of paper work, a urine screen, seeing his nurse practitioner first and then finally, the doctor. My counselor had me scared silly that he would be 'so tough' and 'not receptive' but that could not have been further from the truth! My husband went with me and I kept having to ask him after the appointment, "Are you sure I am not dreaming this?" The doctor was astonished at the amount of damage that my neck has. He was extremely empathetic. He also treated me as an equal human being and did not talk over me, something so many doctors will do if for no other reason than to get you in and out in that fifteen minute space they reserve for you. He explained we will start with my biggest 'hot spot', my neck, and go from there. He was in complete agreement about getting off the Suboxone and so we changed to a medication that is both easy on my stomach, is not a narcotic but acts on the brain in the same way (without the drugged up effect). I would start that in tandem with weaning from the Suboxone. He also explained that my surgeon... indeed the best in town... would do a good job but the surgery would help the stenosis but likely not the neck. He knew I had epidural blocks but informed me there was another procedure that was better and we could do a trial run and if that seemed to help then proceed with more. I felt such a sense of relief and empowerment. We will be filing a complaint on my other doctor for bullying me into signing a release and using a reason that is an outright lie.

It has been two weeks since I first saw my new pain management doctor. In that two weeks I have had better pain control than I have in three years. Am I pain free? No, and until there is a cure for fibromyalgia, I never will be. I am still having issues with insomnia, IBS, anxiety and pretty much all the other issues that go along with fibro. It does bear mentioning my headaches have eased up a great deal but I believe that is because I have substantially reduced my diet soda intake. I have heard so many bad things about aspartame over the years, I decided to try and reduce my intake. It appears to have worked because the one day I upped my soda intake to what I normally would have drunk before, I got a bad headache!

For twenty years I have hurt, spent sleepless nights, been to doctor after doctor, some who believe fibro is 'all in the patients head' or it depression/anxiety and some who know it is real but are frustrated because they do not know what causes it or what can be done for it besides the usual: medication, rest, diet, homeopathic remedies, etc. Luckily most doctors worth their weight stand firm: fibromyalgia is a cruel and unforgiving condition. I have on far too many occasions been at the mercy of my gut. I have been judged both by those who know me and even supposedly love me and in many cases by people before they have even met me. I now have to have my husband fill in my sentences for me much of the time. I am the "uh, uh, um, um" girl because every third word seems to be uh or um. Yet I can pour words on a keyboard like the stuttering country singer that sings like a charm as soon as the banjo plays. It takes me three times long to do anything: get ready, cook, go shopping, etc. I never thought I would be totally disabled in my mid-forties! I wanted a career. I wanted to be able to drive to work each day, gripe about my job, look forward to weekends and earn my paycheck just like everyone else. I had plans for myself by the time I would be turning fifty years old. Sadly, a force I cannot reckon with has gotten in the way. I was going to be that eccentric, bohemian, artsy lady that wears colorful clothing and creates things. I was going to go to the beach and still be riding roller coasters well into my sixties... hands in the air! I finally had my dream come true! I lost my weight! However, I am so fatigued by this beast known as fibromyalgia I fear what I would feel like if I were still twice the woman I once was. Now I will need a scooter if I stand a chance to get around any amusement park to even last eight hours. Traveling? I have to load up on ½ a bottle of Imodium and never mind what that stuff might be doing to me... taking four to five times the recommended dosage. Nonetheless, if I want to go somewhere, I have got to make sure the IBS does not go into overdrive. When a normal person has had a long, tiring day, they are wiped out and tired. They sack out on the couch or go to bed and wake up refreshed. When I over-do it, I can barely walk. I feel like every inch of me has been beat with a baseball bat. I walk like a hunched over ninety year old on hot coals. I at many times fall asleep but am in so much pain I wake up in the night... body throbbing... and hurt too much to sleep anymore. I am usually in a flare for a week. Having fibromyalgia feels like a pack of elephants have run over you.... after a gaggle of five year old children used you as a human piñata. Alas, I have hope! Until I draw my last breathe on earth, I will have hope. In spring of 2012 I started a blog called "Hitting the Wall" http://hittingthewall.paulglover.net/ . This blog is a true labor of love to me and has grown in readership of up to 2000 readers a month. I also make hand-made greeting cards and am trying my hand at starting my own (very) small hand-made greeting card company featuring a line called, "Fibro Care, Fibro Share" which sends a warmhearted hug or a fact about fibro. Albeit I am a bit cynical- often saying when middle aged, rich white men start getting fibro they will truly seek a cure. All the same, I have seen progress in twenty years. It has gone from scribbling on a prescription pad to numerous therapies and procedures including holistic treatments like diet, tai chi, meditation, counseling and so much more. For the tangible issues in my neck I have the surgical option if I desire. Yes, fibromyalgia sadly does dictate my life. Even sadder I hate the way it weighs my husband down. This man has made so many sacrifices for me, without complaint. Fibro has required me to give up... or as I should say... tweak many of my dreams. What caused this cruel and unforgiving malady? Was I born with the predisposition to it? Studies have shown it is hereditary. My Mother and Father both had much physical pain in their lives. My Mother's drinking did and still does have a huge effect on many of my emotional issues. I developed costochondritis many years before I was diagnosed with fibro. In my opinion it was in a large part due to my chicken pox because I was never the same after having this illness. I will probably never know why I have fibromyalgia. Nonetheless, I am here and I have lived this bumpy, crazy and wild ride for twenty years. My dream is to live to see a cure found for this horrendous condition. However, if I do not, I just want some peace, a little happiness and as many good experiences in whatever capacity I can get them in along the way. Oh, and one more thing and possibly the most important, I want to leave the world a little bit better than it was before I was here.

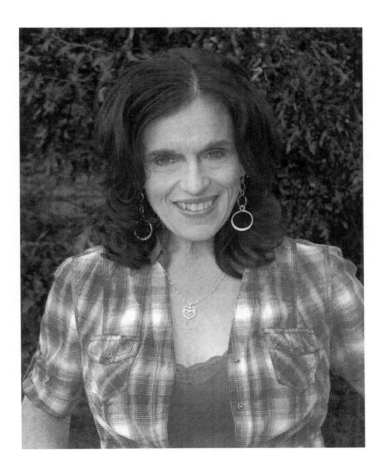

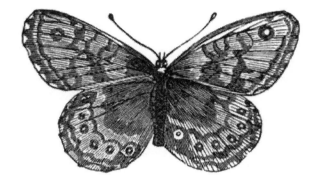

Exhausted and Thankful

By Dawn Lewis

My Name is Dawn and I am 41 years old. I am married, have a teenage daughter and four dogs. I live in Arkansas in a very small town .

I had a good childhood, with one sister and parents who are still married. We are a very close family, including cousins who are more like siblings. My maternal grandmother had some health issues, with early onset RA (Rheumatoid Arthritis), among blood problems and other things, and died at the young age of fifty-nine. My mom and two of my cousins have fibromyalgia. My mom has a great deal of pain, although she is able to work full-time, and one of my cousins has been able to maintain a good deal of activity.

I was diagnosed at 17 with MVP (Mitral Valve Prolapse) and had terrible migraines during my teens. I have scoliosis as well, but other than that have had no serious illnesses. When I was in my late thirties I began having a great deal of neck stiffness and pain, shoulder pain, and headaches. I went to my GP and requested an RA test, given my grandmother's history. My RA factor was slightly high so I was referred to a rheumatologist, who did blood work to rule out anything else and finally

88

*diagnosed me with fibromyalgia. I had not had any physical
trauma, but had experienced some emotional trauma and a
great deal of stress due to some difficult experiences for many
years prior, beginning in my 20's when I was in an abusive
marriage. I feel that for me the fibro was triggered by years of
the trauma, stress, and grief.*

*I worked full time for many years; used to go camping, hiking,
swimming, and spent a lot of time with my sister, cousins, and
their children. I was the "cool" aunt that stayed up late with
the kids and that the teenagers could relate to. Now, with the
fibro, I can't do all of those activities, or anything requiring
physical strength and stamina. I stay at home- unable to work
due to pain, fatigue, fog, and depression. I also deal with many
other common fibro symptoms, such as memory loss, sleep
disturbances, body temperature regulation issues, and nausea,
to name just a few. Though I am not completely disabled I still
have difficulty with mobility at times and very low energy
levels. I am just thankful to be able to still care for myself, and
to cook and clean and shop.*

*I have a sixteen year old daughter from a previous marriage.
My current husband and I have been married for ten years,
and unfortunately have never been able to have children
together. We do however have four dogs who we love, and
they are kind of our kids. My husband and the rest of my*

family are very understanding and don't get upset or resentful when I am not able to do all of the activities I used to. I am grateful for this, however the constant pain and other issues still make for mental and emotional exhaustion most of the time.

I like to read and watch tv, and play some computer games and puzzles. I like spending time on Facebook where I belong to an online support group for fibromyalgia. I enjoy cooking- though cleaning up the mess is another story. I am currently working on my certification for dog behavior and training- so that I can better care for our dogs.

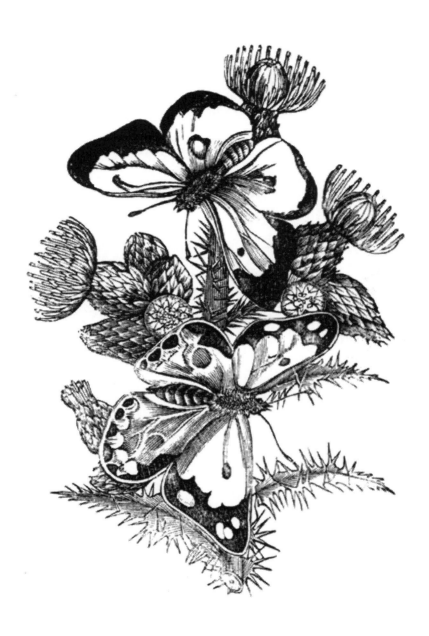

My Foggy Brain... My Journey... My Life

By Tamiko Arbuckle

When you wake up in the morning, what is the first thing that comes to mind? For me, it's... "What hurts? Can I move? Will I be able to get out of bed? Is my brain functioning?" After that, I lay there for a while slowly moving from my toes to my forehead to assess my pain level and mentally prepare myself for the day to come. It wasn't always like this...

Let me introduce myself. My name is Tamiko and I live with Fibromyalgia, Major Depression, Anxiety, ADD, Essential Tremor, and honestly? I could go on, but I am not here to tell you about all my medical issues. I was asked to contribute to this book and share my story... my journey with Fibromyalgia. So! Sit back, relax and hopefully while you read my story; you will smile and even possibly laugh a little bit. My life is here for your reading entertainment (and it's possibly the only time I will ever hope someone laughs at me!).

My own personal disclaimer... I'm sure like many of you reading this, your ability to remember things is not as good as you'd like it to be. Half the time I don't know if it is an actual memory I experienced or a memory from a dream I had at one point. That is probably the most frustrating feeling for me... The number of times someone says to me, "remember when... ?" or when I am sharing an experience I had (or think I had) and half way through the story my mind just draws a blank. I say all this because I am about to tell you my story. It's what I remember and Lord knows my memory fails me on a daily basis!

When I look back over the last four decades (honestly, has it really been that long?), I think of the different phases I have lived through... my childhood (mostly amazing until my angst-filled teen years), my 20's and 30's (marriage, children, fish, dog, buying our first house, cars etc. not necessarily in that order), my pre-FMS crazy working years and now to my post-FMS diagnosis years. No doubt about it, it's been one heck of a roller coaster ride over the decades! I don't believe people that end up with a diagnosis like Fibromyalgia have lived a relaxed, trouble-free life. I believe you have to work really hard to break your body and end up in this kind of pain!

Growing up, I was a feisty, rebellious child who questioned and challenged everything (and I mean everything! Rules? What rules?). Now that I have had the privilege of being a parent, I feel like I should start and end every day with a five-minute call to my folks apologizing to them for all the heartache I caused over the years. It would go something like this:

...ring... ring... ring

My dad (because my mom basically never answers the phone): *"hello?"*

Me: *"Hi dad!"*

My dad: (laughing… he always laughs when he hears it's me on the phone, it makes me smile every time) *"Hey! Is that the mother of my grand-children?"*

Me: *"I'm calling to apologize again for driving you to the brink of insanity during my young adult life. I know I caused you to worry excessively. Thank you for not giving up on me!"*

My dad: *"CHIZUKO!!! Your daughter is on the phone again…"* (Now I hear my folks bickering as my dad hangs up and my mom picks up.)

My mom: *"hello? Who is this?"*

Me: *"Mom… it's me."*

My mom: *"huh? I can't hear you, who is this!"*

Me: *"Mom… it's me! I was just calling again to apologize…"*

My mom: (cutting me off) *"Oh my God! Don't be silly!"* (I am editing what she'd actually say so you don't think badly of this wonderful woman I call my mom).

Me: *"Okay mom, tell dad I love him… I love you and I'll talk to you again in the morning!"*

From a toddler until the day I moved out I gave my parents hell. I thank the Lord every day for blessing me with parents who loved me unconditionally and had endless amounts of patience and forgiveness.

As a child, I strived for independence at a young age. I loved school until I moved in the middle of 9th grade. I transferred from a very small junior high in Oregon where I had finally reached the top of the class to a pretty big high school in Palo Alto, CA where I was once again at the bottom. I found myself in a new school where I knew no one, in one of the wealthiest cities in the area... hundreds of miles from all my friends. Let's just say my rebelliousness reached an all time high. I couldn't, or better said... I *didn't know how* to handle the changes. At 15, after realizing I wasn't going to succeed in regular school, I started independent studies and got a job. I graduated early and started working full-time.

The feeling of working, setting goals, meeting deadlines and ultimately advancing in my career became very important to me. I was learning what it meant to be responsible and the feeling of accountability for my every day activities... and at the end of the day, the pride I felt in my results drove me to want to work harder.

At a certain point, it wasn't the advancement I was looking for but the feeling of accomplishment and value that I added to the organization. As I continued to work harder and harder and take on more and more responsibility, my hours significantly increased along with my stress. At the height of all this, I was working 16+ hours a day (at least 6 days a week), eating all my meals in the office and getting very little sleep. When my children were born, I worked up until I went into labor and went back to work just weeks after they were born. For close to two decades, my work life completely consumed my time and energy. My personal life was non-existent or completely out-of-control. My ability to balance my work and home life was a constant challenge...I felt like a success at work and a failure at home.

And then one tragedy hit after another... first a very close friend of mine was killed in an accident, then my grandmother passed away, followed by my aunt and then my uncle and then my godmother and then an aunt... and it just kept going. The sadness was overwhelming and my ability to recover became more and more difficult. We were traveling to hospitals and funerals and with the amount of hours I had been working, keeping up with everything just became too much.

One day, while playing with my dog Tani outside I felt my back go out. It was at that point my body made a decision it was no longer going to support my lifestyle. Either I make a change willingly or it was going to force a change. I bet you can guess what happened.

I ended up on the couch, where I remained for weeks unable to move. Days passed without me knowing what was going on. I was on so much pain medication that the house could have burned down and I would have slept through it (or not even realized I was about to go up in smoke!). My family still remembers the days when they would laugh at me because I appeared so high (Ummmm... I can't really sugar coat that, I was actually pretty high!). Apparently conversations with me at that time were rather amusing. I just have to believe them... I remember... well, I remember absolutely none of those conversations. This is where my journey with medication and doctors began.

I was in and out of the doctor's office for four years before I was finally diagnosed with Fibromyalgia. The only solution I kept hearing for four years was a prescription of pain pills. When one stopped working I would move to the next one. With all the medical research and advances that have been made, not one of those doctor appointments ended with anything other than a lot of frustration and a new prescription. Each prescription had side effects that impacted my ability to get back to a normal way of life. It may have numbed the pain, but it also numbed my brain (did you catch that rhyme I just did?). So even though I was no longer working those crazy hours at work, I was still not available for my family. Not because of my job, but because I was in this drug induced state every day and night.

The first diagnosis I received was Degenerative Disc disease. It was good to get a name for the pain I was experiencing, but it just didn't explain everything that was going on. The meds that were prescribed were horrible, I remember one of them gave me blurry vision (that was fun thinking I was going blind).

I was not just experiencing back pain though. I was having a really hard time remembering things… like driving in the car and forgetting where I was or where I was going… or how about losing everything (over and over again!)… how to do basic every day stuff… and worst of all… at work, where I had excelled my entire career, I was suffering. It was taking me ten times longer to accomplish what I would do without any thought. My pain was no longer just in my back it was moving all over the place. I was having a hard time walking. I couldn't be touched; I felt like my whole body was one exposed nerve… and let's just talk about my inability to sleep. Sleep was my enemy at night… and the more frustrated I got, the harder it became. My neighbor friend still talks about it… no matter what time he came home at night or left in the morning, the light was always on at my house and I was up. On the flip side of that… Even though I couldn't sleep, I was exhausted. <u>ALL</u> of the time. No energy for anyone or anything.

I felt like I was crazy. My depression was just getting worse and worse and my anxiety was at an all-time high. I would keep going to the doctor for one reason or another and each time my doctor would look at me with that look. You know what I'm talking about... the "look". The one that says, "*I am really trying to help you, but nothing is wrong with you so I'm going to try my best to be empathetic and prescribe something to make you go away.*" That look. More drugs. I left many doctor appointments holding on to my emotions by a thread until I got to my car. Once I shut that car door... the emotional floodgates opened up and I was a wreck. Some of those appointments I wasn't able to keep it together, I just lost it in front of the doctor, my frustration getting the best (or worst) of me. Those are the moments I cherished... my doctor looking at me as if she was deciding whether or not she needed to call in a psychiatrist for support. Me feeling completely hopeless and wondering whether or not something is wrong with me... like is this stuff real or is it all in my head? No one wants to feel like a basket case... especially those of us who were raised and grew up as strong, independent women! I mean I can literally count on one (maybe one and a half) hands the number of times I actually saw my mother cry.

So one day, I was really feeling like crap and I pushed myself to, once again, make an appointment. My doctor was out so I saw a different doctor who then referred me to the Rheumatology department. In a twenty-minute appointment my life changed. The doctor diagnosed me with Fibromyalgia... just like that. He had never seen me before. He asked me several questions, that I'm sure if you are reading this, you are familiar with. How long had I been in pain? Where was the pain? Followed by him asking me to stand up while he proceeded to push all the "tender points" in my body until I was literally crying my eyes out and couldn't hold myself up any longer. I was a winner... I felt pain in every tender point. Twenty minutes later he says to me, "You have Fibromyalgia." I mean, he literally said it to me like he was diagnosing me with a cold. He really didn't understand the magnitude with which this message came to me. To him it was no big deal. To me it was as if he told me I won the lottery... only without the jumping up and down, and of course there was no money at the end of that winning ticket!

I finally had a name... Fibromyalgia. Fi-bro-my-al-gia. What?

At first I thought my prayers were answered. That bubble was burst real soon! I realized very quickly, even with a diagnosis, there was no cure... no solution. I started reading everything I could get my hands on. At that point, there wasn't a ton of information out there. I read book after book and then while doing research online, I discovered all these blogs. I was not alone. There were other people out there who had gone through the same thing as me. Except after reading through a lot of the blogs, I felt worse. Everyone was sharing all their feelings around the pain, frustration and a whole lot of hopelessness. I really started to think my life was over.

I was in a dark place. Literally. I kept the blinds drawn in my bedroom and I stayed in that dark room for many days and weeks. I remember I couldn't walk, I couldn't shower myself, I couldn't do anything on my own. I would try and sit down for dinner with my family and half way down the hallway to the dinner table I would just break down in tears. The pain was unbearable. My husband would turn me around and help me back in bed. I missed the soccer games, the school and family activities, the parenting. I was no longer living in the real world. I was in some alternate universe where all I saw was the four walls in my room, a ton of TV and, I played a lot of Facebook games (Farmville anyone?).

I needed an outlet. I needed a way to get rid of all the crap in my head and the emotions I was feeling. I decided to start my own blog, just for myself. I didn't share it with anyone I knew. I didn't want people close to me to read stuff that was so painfully personal to me. I just started writing. At the same time, I joined the Twitter world. I found this amazing community of people, men and women, young and old, from Sweden to the UK to Canada to all the states in the U.S... this stuff is not picky, it will attack anyone... at any time. I started to tweet and share my thoughts, my pain and bits and pieces of my life. I shared information that I thought would help people. I started to share my blog. I found my voice and I found a community that understood and supported me.

This was my turning point. I realized I was not alone, and more importantly I realized that there _was_ life with Fibromyalgia. I got more aggressive with my doctors and I was finally admitted into the pain programs at Kaiser. I started to learn how to cope and manage my pain.

I have been asked a lot over the years how I cope with chronic pain (physical and mental)... I have many answers to that question. Laughter... laughter is a huge way to kill the evils of pain. Getting out and spending time with my family and friends, the folks that have been there for me through this long journey. They may not truly understand what it's like to live with all the stuff I struggle with, but they certainly have been there to make me laugh. I have learned I don't always have to leave my house to "get out". Sometimes just getting out of bed and out of my bedroom is enough. That's the thing... the people that I surround myself with understand my limitations. It's important to keep positive, uplifting folks around you... especially if they make you laugh!

Exercise... we all hate it. If we haven't done it in a long time, it's painful to start. For me, it's the difference between flaring 24/7 and flaring a few days here and there. I believe it is the gentle movement that wakes your body up. It's a time when you are in control and you are telling the pain to go away (or you can use more harsh words than "go away", if you'd like... I do). The key for me is "gentle" movement. Yoga, Tai Chi, Qigong, Feldenkreis, stretching and walking are the types of exercise I have tried and have helped me. I have even completed a couple 5K's (walking, of course, let's not get too crazy here)!! For me, my depression and anxiety are as bad as my Fibromyalgia; even worse now that I have learned how to manage my pain better... exercise is key to better mental health for me.

Eating the right foods... I struggle with this every day. Food makes a huge difference for me, not only because of the pain, but I also suffer from IBS and GERD. If one thing is exacerbated than the pain jumps right in there to make sure it gets its proper attention. I have to stay away from the food that triggers a bad reaction in my body... basically I have had to learn to live without a lot of really yummy food. If I stray even a little, I suffer. It is the true definition of *consequences* (Darn those consequences!!).

There is always that balance that has to be kept between pain management, digestive health, and mental health... the worst of all three come out to play when there's stress. So keeping my stress down is critical. Meditation, prayer, and a lot of lessons I learned from cognitive behavioral therapy help keep me sane. Well, most of the time anyway. No one's perfect. If you believe you have to be perfect, stress will be your best friend forever.

There was a time when I went 6 months without driving. Actually there was a period of years where I didn't drive... except maybe down the street when absolutely necessary. There was a long period of time when I walked with a cane... a very long time. There was also a time when I used a wheelchair. I wasn't able to shower without my husband washing my hair and helping me bathe myself. I couldn't go up and down stairs. I couldn't ride in the car for long periods of time. I call this my "dependent" period.

During that "dependent" period, I was on so many prescription pills that I had to keep getting bigger and bigger pillboxes. I had to get one that I could separate my morning, afternoon and evening pills. One day I decided to just stop the madness. I never liked taking pills and I felt like the side effects were far worse than the benefit. When I finally made the decision to stop the meds I had been suicidal for months. Every day all I thought about was if I was dead, there would be no more pain, no more suffering, no more sadness... and no more burden on those around me. I played the scenarios out in my head, what it would look like with me gone. My family moving on with their lives without me... I could no longer see beyond the black and grey clouds that constantly enveloped me. I was desperate. I finally looked at my husband one night, while in tears (again) and we decided together that it was time to do something drastic. I called my doctor and we agreed on a plan to taper off everything. The best decision I would ever make.

It has been almost two years now and I will never (at least I hope I never) rely on medication to manage my pain long-term again. I ended up going back on anti-depressants... I am not sure I can ever live without them... and every once in awhile I will take something to help the pain and I am okay with this.

I am still dependent on my husband, he's my rock, my best friend and at times he is still my caretaker. Thankfully, I am not in that "dependent" period anymore. I am driving. I am finishing 5K's, I am more self-sufficient, I am a healthier person overall. I am living.

Every day is not a good day. There will always be bad days. I know it's my choice how I fight back and whether or not I fight to live a healthy and happy life. I am blessed that I don't have anything life-threatening. What I have is a reminder... a reminder that if I want to feel alive, I need to choose a lifestyle that brings me joy and gives me the freedom to live well. I know I need to make choices that will result in less pain. The pain never goes away, but it doesn't have to be debilitating every minute and every hour of every day.

I have had my blog for almost four years now. I focused my blog around hope and how to live with Fibromyalgia, with Major Depression, with ADD... and a whole host of other things that keep joining the party of diseases and syndromes that seem to enjoy being hosted by my body. The last diagnosis being Essential Tremor... that's a fun one! I go back and forth on whether or not to continue with my blog... for me, it has served its purpose. It saved me when I thought no one understood what I was going through. It lifted my spirits when people left comments telling me they felt the same way and thanked me for sharing... it helped my family and friends better understand my pain and how to respond to my changed life. When I think about taking my blog down, my husband is the first one to say "NO!". He reminds me that no matter how I am feeling today, people still visit it for information, and to see that there is someone out there who understands. So, for now, it's there. And it's the reason why I was given this opportunity to share my journey with you.

I hope that my story has given you hope. You can stop by and visit me anytime at the following URL:

http://myfoggybrain.com/

Gentle hugz! Stay cool and live your life to the fullest… tomorrow is not promised, but take the opportunity today to make it a great day.

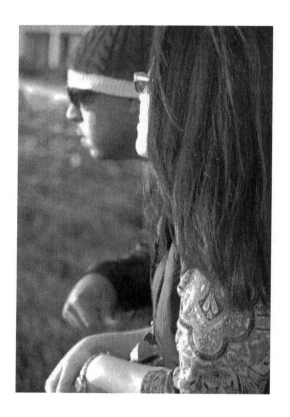

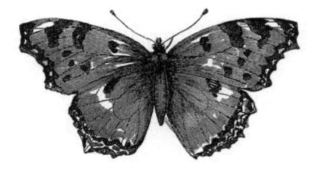

The Fibromonster

By Vanessa McCutcheon

My name is Vanessa. I was diagnosed with (I call it) the fibromonster in 2011. Looking back, and most of us know about hindsight, I wonder just how long I really had been fighting it. I live in the northwestern part of South Carolina and have been a Registered Nurse for 18 years. At age 59 I was a little older than the average age for a fibromyalgia diagnosis. I was working with a wonderful hospice care organization providing home care and completely loving my job. I worked long hours and almost always carried a larger than normal patient case load. I also did some of the precept services for new employees and supervision for LPNs. It was hard work, mentally and often physically, long hours and on call nights and weekends, demanding as in all the paperwork had to be on time, correct and meeting federal guidelines and it was often heartbreaking. But I loved it, and I was good at it, not everyone can say that. But I pushed and denied until I reached the point that I could not go another day.

I was a healthy kid. I did have what is called "growing pains" in my legs as a child. I grew up spending most of my time outside or reading. I hated school but loved college, imagine that. Later as an adult I developed osteoarthritis, which ran strongly in my mother's family.

I had never known anyone with fibromyalgia; I don't remember it being taught in the curriculum in college. I looked it up in my textbooks which I have held onto all these years and it was barely mentioned and no indication I had ever noticed it was in there. Really the first contact I ever had with fibromyalgia was when I had a patient and the caregiver told me they could not pull and lift on the patient because they had it. Since I had no knowledge of how devastating fibro can be, I had no understanding or sympathy for their situation. What is it they say about payback?

Sometime in 2008 or 2009 I began having weird, brief, transient periods of pain. I finally went to my Dr. and the only way I could describe what I was experiencing was to tell him to picture a slowly moving disco ball...you know the ones with the blinking lights, revolving slowly...and wherever on my body the light fell, I had brief pain until the light blinked off....then again and again... He looked at me and asked what I had been smoking...but he believed me. The pain varied in intensity, sometimes sharp and stabbing, sometimes a dull ache, sometimes a combination. I also was very tired. He did some blood work and my vitamin D was borderline low. He decided I had Chronic Fatigue Syndrome and treated me with high dose D supplements. Life went on the pain continued but not to a point that OTC s couldn't take the edge off for a while, but it escalated. I kept denying and pushing myself until I was using Demerol to help with the pain (I had it left over from having my tonsils removed). I began reading everything I could find on CFS and noticed that usually fibromyalgia was discussed in the same book or article. I compared symptoms then found a tender/pressure point map for fibromyalgia and discovered I had all of them. Things progressed until I was beyond exhausted, I was having a very difficult time climbing steps or stairs, could not tolerate too hot or too cold temperatures. I began having nausea just out of the blue, I was having a very hard time taking a deep breath, like when you yawn but can't yawn deeply enough to feel satisfied. My patients thought I was sleepy, very embarrassing, but I guess it is what is called air hunger; I felt like I was starving for air.

I think it was a Tuesday. I went in to work, had to climb a flight of stairs. By the time I made it to my desk I was about to collapse from pain and exhaustion. I told my supervisor I had to go see my doctor. I was panting and had tears streaming *down my face, I wasn't crying but have you ever noticed how when you yawn your eyes sometime water...it is like that. I have not worked since. When my doctor walked in the room I was having to brace myself against the wall to draw in a deep breath. I still get that air hunger when I'm in a stressful situation.*

I also saw a rheumatologist and after 3-4 visits he diagnosed the fibromonster. He put me on Cymbalta and that cost me about three months of memories... bad stuff for me. The pain doctor that I was sent to thought it was funny that the Cymbalta messed with my head. He started asking questions like if I was promiscuous! He also talked about how he was going to have to try dating older women (he was in his early 40s) because the younger women he had been dating 'just didn't get it.' I did get it... and I didn't go back. No, I didn't report it, but I still think about it.

I take extended release morphine and Tramadol for pain control, I found a spray topical pain relief that really helps, works for muscle and joint pain. I use Zanaflex for muscle spasms and take a handful of supplements, no joke! Plus stuff for sleep, stuff for nausea, stuff for shortness of breath, or tension, stuff for blood clot prevention.

I go very few places and see very few people. Going to the grocery store is dreaded; I do that early when my energy is at its best. One time when I HAD to do several errands, on a Saturday, my legs were hurting, I had nausea, and had a granddaughter with me and had to stop at the grocery I used my handicapped placard. I also had my son, to drive for me, and his friend. When we came out someone had left an ugly note on my car that they were 70% handicapped and never used Handicapped parking. I only use it if I'm hurting bad but I guess since my disability isn't visually obvious, people think its cheating to use it.

I'm happy here at home but do get lonely at times. We, my husband and I, and before fibro, often met with friends to cook out, pot-luck or watch football and we would meet friends for a drink. I too often found that my unpredictable nausea kept popping up so I began to more and more often stay home. Now we are not invited out anymore. Right after I was put out of work my friends from there would call me to meet them for lunch but the same thing...I cancelled till they stopped calling too.

About 6-7 years ago, when I was single, I was spending Friday and Saturday evenings ballroom dancing nonstop for 5-6 hours each day. During the week after work I walked 3 miles, every day, and worked out on one of those machines Chuck Norris sells....can't remember the name. Now there are days that I can barely walk outside, none that I walk without pain. For a while I used a cane as my balance is very poor and unstable but that caused extra pain in my entire arm from my hands to my upper back, so I rarely use it now but find there are times I wish I had it. I do still try to exercise. Our home is in the country and we have almost 2 acres. When my husband is home we walk the boundaries when I'm able. He pushes me some days that I feel bad, to try. I'm glad he does but there are those days that nothing takes the pain away enough.

My symptoms are pain, mostly in my rt. hip, buttock, and even my outer "lady parts." (I never would have thought about pain in the buttock being real til now- but totally never thought about fibro attacking my "lady parts!"), thigh, calf, and foot. My right foot is never free of pain. I also hurt in my left arm, shoulder to hand, my back, and I have frequent headaches. All of these sites hurt almost nonstop day and night to some degree. Other areas join in whenever they feel the need to remind me they are there and want me to know.

I have nausea almost daily from mild to dry heaves. My vision has blurred. I have the most annoying ringing in my ears. The fatigue is so bad that some days it feels like I haven't slept at all. I have pretty severe dizziness upon standing at times. There are days when the pain and fatigue are so bad I only move around my home, from bed to couch. Plus I'm dreaming. I have not remembered dreaming for years, I do now. The fibro fog is worse some times more than others. The most annoying part of it for me is that sometimes when I do have to drive I get what I call tunnel vision. It seems like the street or road just stretches out forever and at the same time things, other cars, signs, buildings, roads or streets are flying toward me. Also...I have had a few occasions that I suddenly feel lost...nothing looks familiar...that is frightening! Thankfully it only lasts for a very brief time but I worry that the next time....what if? Now my husband does all the driving and nearly all the time I panic to some degree. Once it was so bad that I had the air hunger with tears rolling. He was going 40mph but it felt like he was going 75-80. Now when I MUST go out I usually go ahead and take a tranquilizer and that takes the edge off. I drive only short distances, 2-4 miles, and only if there is no choice. The last time I tried to drive, the road was stretched out and everything was racing toward me... I turned around and came home.

I now fill my time reading, I do editing and proof reading (free of charge) for a couple of fiction writers. I also make barrettes for mostly my granddaughters, but I have a daughter that teaches special needs children and she takes some to school with her sometimes. For a while I created the most beautiful Easter eggs, turning them into animals or with intricate designs but obviously have problems with some fine motor skills as I just can't do those any more. We are attempting to garden. I would love to be able to grow some of our food, and that project is going slowly.

When I lost my job, I lost my medical insurance as well. My husband's employer doesn't offer insurance so everything is self-pay. That makes it hard. Thankfully we don't have much debt but income is limited.

One of the most trying experiences and emotionally painful is telling someone why I am "sick." So many times the response is "well I must have that too; my arm has been just killing me." Or "I am tired all the time I wonder if I have that" the best one so far has been "But, that doesn't kill you does it?" It's like forget that everything you know as your day to day life has been stolen, transformed, ripped apart, beat up and stomped on then smashed together and returned to you as an existence you don't even recognize much less want or like, or know how to survive, but it's supposed to be ok since it won't kill you. They have no way of knowing, of course, that there have been a few times that that almost would have not been a true statement.

So it's just me, my husband of 3 years, my cat, and 7 chickens. Our kids are grown. The grands visit occasionally. But too often gramma feels bad. I hate for that to be their memories of me as I have wonderful memories of being with my grandmother. I always do my best to plan and do something special with them. We cook and garden. I want so badly for them to be involved in nature and have some knowledge of how things grow. Each year they plant something, watch it grow, then gather and eat it. That is priceless.

I am so thankful that I found an online Fibromyalgia Forum. There, nobody says, "Well that won't kill you." The members know, understand what fibromyalgia takes from you. That has been one of the best things I have found to help cope with losses I have had, simple acceptance and understanding.

I have also learned some important lessons about how to deal with life with this monster, so I shall end with those:

1. If you can, do it now. (There is no guarantee you will feel better later, tomorrow, next week or ever.)

2. This may be your best day, find some pleasure. (There is no guarantee you will feel better later, tomorrow, next week or ever.)

3. If someone offers to do it for you, let them. ~this may be your best day, letting them do it for you may give you the time to do something pleasurable, like take a nap~(There is no guarantee you will feel better later, tomorrow, next week or ever.)

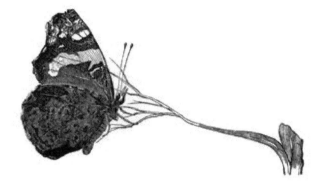

Outside Looking In

By Connie Papp

The silence outside is a welcome respite

contrasting the thoughts colliding and crashing

relentlessly, unacknowledged

and forgotten

The foggy facade envelops in a blanket of blackness

conceding misjudgment, misinterpretation and missteps

to ensue

In sly, sadistic synchronicity the pain rages

To echo in kind

A greedy ever present reminder demanding attention

never to be stifled

Minute by minute, day after unyielding day

with no reprieve….precious time pilfered

Held hostage inside the shell of the old me

grieving for the days my body was able

Some would have given up long ago

waiving their white flag soaked in salty, tortured tears

But....we go on

Living not the life in our dreams, but life

as it is now

Piercing the pain and fog momentarily; your whispers

of compassion reminding me, you are here,

you are alive and above all else

...you are loved

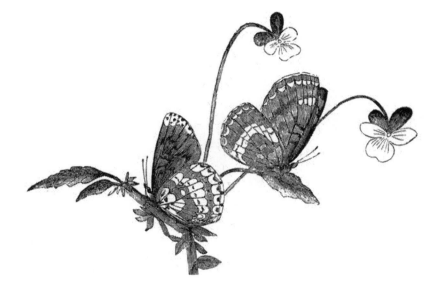

Making it Work

By Susan Sunny Johnson

My name is Susan but as a kid I was given the nickname "Sunny" because of my "sunny disposition." I am 55 years old and live in a small town in northwest Florida. I have 3 brothers and had a difficult childhood. My parents were considered affluent in our small town, and if you have ever lived in a small town you know that can make life difficult for a shy teenager. Truthfully they probably should have stayed single and neither were really meant to be parents. That being said, I believe they did the best they could.

There was always a lot of stress in our household and I believe the first onset of fibromyalgia began as depression and stomach problems at about 8 or 9 years old. My parents were going through a divorce (their first of 3) and the stress in our household was so thick you could cut it with a knife, and there was a lot of violence as well. There was an eleven year age difference between my parents, and my father drank when he was stressed. My mother was all about appearances, so to the outside world we were the perfect family, but behind closed doors it was a completely different story.

126

Throughout my childhood my parents fought with my fraternal grandparents over our religious upbringing. Many times I remember being taken off of our front porch by my grandparents while my mother was upstairs getting ready for church. She would come downstairs to take us to church and we would be gone. It was always a war zone on Sundays, but not all of my memories are bad. I have many good memories too, such as summer camp and Sunday dinners at my grandmother's, and I always had someone to play with growing up. Being the only girl had its advantages at times. I didn't ever have to wear hand-me-down clothes, and we had a housekeeper/nanny who loved me to the moon and back and taught me all of the arts of being a woman. She taught me how to run a home and cook, how to do laundry properly and iron.

I was very shy and withdrawn, and did not make friends easily. I was also considered "beautiful," the kind of child who should have been in pageants and on stage, but my shyness and propensity for hysteria prevented me from participating in these kinds of activities. Looking back now, I believe I suffered from some form of depression even before my teens. I basically had no self-esteem because my father told me repeatedly that girls were not the same as boys and did not have the abilities that boys did. When I expressed a desire to be either an architect or an attorney when I grew up, my dad told me that I was not smart enough and that those were men's jobs. Girls should be teachers or nurses- this is what I was told, so I became a teacher. It was clear that my father was disappointed that his first-born was a girl.

My mother sent me to boarding school my junior year in high school because of the tension between my father and me. We could not get along and there was even violence between us. When I returned I had found my voice and was able to stand up to him. He and my mom had divorced for the final time, so he bought me a car in exchange for my living with him and helping him with my brothers. I was under no rules, so I agreed. My senior year I went back to my local high school and was talked into entering a local county pageant, and I won. It was the beginning of more trouble though; all of the girls hated the "interloper," and the boys were intimidated, so my senior year ended up being very lonely.

I was not a healthy child, with frequent ear and throat infections. In the third grade I had my appendix removed and in the sixth grade had my tonsils out. I was getting fevers that were unexplained and after I started my menstrual cycle I had horrible cramps and heavy bleeding. I missed a lot of school during childhood because of illness, and as a result I changed schools three times. I was the kid who was always sick and stayed up late with a flashlight so I could read under the covers. I loved books about horses or dogs and devoured any I could get my hands on. Books were my friends- they never hurt your feelings or made you feel left out. I was just the pretty girl everyone thought had lots of friends, but in reality didn't get invited to parties or sleepovers, so I read- a lot. My room became my sanctuary and the characters in my books were my friends. Was I lonely? Sure, sometimes, but I was more afraid of being the awkward one in a group, so I rarely accepted when I was asked to participate in group activities.

At the age of sixteen I went to a party with a few friends from my neighborhood. It was in the woods behind a boy's house and there was a bonfire. There were a few boys drinking beer and the music was loud, and everyone was laughing and having fun when suddenly from nowhere one boy swooped down on me at a full dead-on run and grabbed me up, running through the woods like a maniac, all the while laughing like he was rescuing me from something horrible... then he tripped and I went flying through the air. I landed on my head and shoulders, and was paralyzed- I could see and hear but not move or speak. Well, being that we were kids at a party where there was drinking, and no one knew what to do, one of the boys carried me into the house and laid me on the bed. I remember laying there until I could eventually move my hands and arms. After a couple of hours I got a ride home, snuck into the house, and never told my parents what had happened. The next day I stayed home claiming a migraine, when in fact was I couldn't turn my head. God only knows the damage I did that night, but I believe that is the main beginning trigger for my symptoms to this day.

According to my family history, of which there is no written record but is passed down by word of mouth, there is a long history of depression, dementia, and anger problems on my father's side of the family. Many on that side have also had OCD and ADD/ADHD. My dad was diagnosed with OCD/ADHD and borderline personality disorder, and he drove us all crazy growing up. We never knew what was going to happen next. In his 60s my dad began using drugs in earnest, and by his late 70s he was addicted to crack cocaine. He died at age 83 of congestive heart failure, dementia, and COPD, all exacerbated by his excessive drug use. I believe he also suffered from depression, though it was undiagnosed.

My oldest brother has the same symptoms as my dad, as well as a history of drug use. In fact all three of my brothers have drug use in their pasts, and my youngest brother also has a history of gambling. The two older ones have both cleaned up their acts and beat the drug problems, and I am very proud of both of them. My middle brother had the worst problem, to the extent that he was unable to work for several years and I ended up with custody of his children for four years. However he has cleaned up and gone back to work, and is raising his kids himself now. My youngest brother is still battling his demons and I pray daily that he will be able to beat back that old devil before it gets him. All three of my brothers struggle with serious anger and self-control issues, and each have violent tempers, but to my knowledge none of them have signs or symptoms of fibromyalgia. Though I love them very much we are not very close.

My symptoms were dormant for many years so when I think of my health, I tend to think in terms of 'before' and 'after.' Before, when my kids were young, I was able to go in twelve directions at once, sleep without drugs and the strongest thing I ever took was an aspirin. I finished my college degree in three years all while raising two small children, and sometimes I marvel at the fact that I survived that at all! We went to ball practice in the afternoons, races on the weekends, church on Sunday, family holidays, and all the while I went to work immediately after graduating. I played softball and was very active with my children in their sports activities.

I should have known it couldn't last forever. That is when my first symptoms really began. My marriage broke up in a brutal fashion and my depression deepened. I attempted suicide. I began to have aches and pains that I couldn't explain and I began to be labeled by family members as a whiner... a quitter. I had become a teacher like my dad wanted me to be, and I hated being in the classroom. Don't get me wrong, I loved the kids and I was good at it, but the restrictiveness was horrendous. I began to know something was really wrong when I would fall asleep during reading groups. No matter what I did, I couldn't stay awake. After the fourth year of classroom work an opportunity came up and I was able to change jobs within the school system to become a grant manager for Single Parents and Parenting Teens as well as Displaced Homemakers. That was right up my alley! I excelled at my work and became happy again! I worked long hours, won numerous awards, traveled to conferences statewide and spoke at conventions. I even remarried. Then one morning I woke up and couldn't get out of bed. I called frantically to my husband and he rushed to my side. He helped me sit up on the side of the bed and rubbed the feeling back into my hands and legs and feet until I could stand. He then helped me into a hot shower. Afterwards, I felt better but I think that was the real beginning for me.

As life progressed, my children grew, my new marriage began to have problems and the financial problems began to get worse. I was having more and more bad days and missing more and more work (thank God for Family Medical Leave!) Friends stopped inviting me to participate in group activities because inevitably I would have to drop out at the last minute anyway and life began to spiral out of control. Then the economy tanked. Pink slips were being handed out like lottery tickets and since I had been working out of field for twenty five years (outside of the classroom and my certified area) my job was dissolved and I was sent to work as a fifth grade teacher an hour away from where I live. The shock was such that I felt betrayed and as if I had had my hair set on fire and put out on the curb to watch it burn. I had done so much good for the school- I couldn't believe it. I only had five more years to full retirement. I had not been in a classroom in so many years that even though I was certified in elementary education, I knew I could not do it. However I packed up and moved to the new school to give it a try. I ended up with a great bunch of kids but I was suddenly thrust into a situation where there were over ninety faculty and staff members, 1800 children and I did not know a single soul. Nor was I offered any help, mentoring or guidance. I struggled and every morning I made the drive to work wondering what it would be like if I just drove off one of the many bridges, or veered into the lane of an oncoming semi. I cried all the way there and all the way home. This lasted six weeks and one night after a really bad day, my husband said "that's it. No more." So the next day I got to work and as I was trying to juggle the heavy fire door open while carrying a crate of books, my heel caught on the threshold and the fire door slammed me from behind, sending me flying across the room. I lay there stunned for several minutes until someone came by and saw my foot sticking out the door like the wicked witch of the west and called for help. I was transported by ambulance and although my hip was not broken or fractured I had a nasty bruise and a mild concussion. I was out for a couple of weeks but happier than I could imagine. So my husband and I made the decision at that point that twenty five years of my life was all they were entitled to. So I filed for my disability based on my bi-polar and Fibromyalgia, and put in my retirement. Yes, I get less money than if I had stuck it out, but I would not have survived it. I had a wonderful Psychiatrist who diagnosed me with severe depression, bi-polar, borderline personality disorder and PTSD after losing the job and being thrust into an unfamiliar setting with no support. I could have sued the district and probably won but I just wanted out- away from the chaos. Life is simpler now, I miss having the structure a job offers me and a place to be every day but I find ways to fill my time.

My symptoms run the gamut. Some are mild, some are horrible but after all these years I can honestly say I am in a kind of remission right now and I thank God for that. If I had to list them it would go something like this, IBS, severe muscle cramps, joint pain, numbness in my hands, feet and limbs. Night sweats- I wake up several times at night wringing wet and frozen from the inside out forcing me to change clothes and sometimes even the sheets on the bed. They are the worst. I also deal with TMJ, neck pain, tingling and burning in my feet and odd places like spots on my arms and legs. Sometimes my skin hurts so bad I can't wear clothes or be touched. There's nausea, constipation, diarrhea, teeth grinding. But worst of all is the fog- the famous fibro fog, and the loss of my command of the English language. I have always prided myself on my vocabulary and use of the English language as well as my ability to write and speak in public. One of my main jobs as a counselor was to write grants and I was very good at it. I facilitated large conferences for hundreds of participants. Now, I am lucky if I can write a check without getting it wrong. And my memory recall- it seems to have abandoned me. In the midst of a conversation I will just forget what I was saying and although I can see the words in my head and feel them on my tongue I can't get them out. It's humiliating for me; I used to stand in front of hundreds of people and give motivational speeches. Now I can't carry on a conversation in the grocery line.

I went to so many doctors, most of whom told me it was in my head, I was tested for every disease known to man until finally they just put me on enough pain and sleep meds to knock down an elephant until one day I realized I had a serious problem. I was addicted. My life in shambles I decided that I had to get clean. So, I quit. I do not recommend the cold turkey method, but for me it was the only choice I had. After two weeks I was drug free. Of course I still don't sleep and I still have the odd pain but my mind is clearing and the fogginess is not as bad.

The first doctor I went to thought I had Lupus, then she said well, it may be Fibromyalgia but there are no tests for that so the best thing to do is live with it. And she sent me home. I began to do my own research after that, I became obsessed with finding doctors who knew more about it, and who believed it to be a real disease until about two years ago when I found a Rheumatologist who did believe me and who treats me as a human being. He did not give me pain meds but gave me low dose Topamax (an anti-seizure drug) that has all but made the majority of my symptoms disappear. How long will it last? I don't know, but for now it is working, and other than the occasional cortisone shot in the neck and shoulder I am holding my own. I can deal with the small stuff. In all it took me around 20 years to find a doctor who took me seriously. I still take Klonopin for anxiety on occasion but mainly I take supplements like a multi vitamin, B12, iron, calcium, protein shakes, and I try to eat a well-balanced diet. I rest when my body tells me too and I know my limits.

As I have discovered in my fibro journey, most people consider me a hypochondriac and their advice is to just get up and move on. Exercise, eat right and get busy. That's the cure, according to the general public, so I try. But when I can't, I just can't. I choose not to be close to my family for many reasons. I have a daughter who does not understand and though I love her and she is my heart we do not have a close relationship. My stepson and I are much closer and he is more understanding. I am still married, but my current husband has developed Hep C so we are in the midst of a pretty unpleasant treatment program for him. He is disabled and I don't know where this will all lead.

Over the years I lost many friends because of this dreadful illness and the depression that accompanies it but I am at a place in my life now that I have stopped asking why and just accepted that it was meant to be. I am no longer angry at my body's betrayal although I will admit to being frustrated at times.

As for friendships, when I retired I maintained two of my work friendships -girlfriends I couldn't get along without- and rekindled an old high school friendship I wouldn't trade for anything. She is my rock! They are all understanding and unwilling to let me wallow when I get too close to the edge of depression. They call me out and push my limits, which is good for me. I love them dearly and just wish I had known them back when I was younger and this all first started. I might not have felt so alone.

My mother does not understand my illness at all and never has. She was always a very strong and forceful woman who ran several businesses. When my step father passed away she suffered a stroke, a heart attack and now has insulin dependent diabetes. She has the beginnings of early onset dementia and is difficult to deal with. Because of things from my childhood, we are not close and do not see one another very often.

Mentally and emotionally this illness has been devastating. I have been institutionalized for severe depression and suicidal thoughts on several occasions. I am on Paxil and Abilify for the depression now and it seems to be helping me to cope, although for a couple of months I tried going drug free and I was a crying mess. Spiritually, I have railed at God asking why me, but now I am at a place in my life where I don't question why anymore, I have accepted this as my lot in life and just have to learn more creative ways to deal with it. Probably the most helpful is rest, and meditation. I have developed some pretty awesome guided meditations that I walk myself through when things are really bad and I can calm down and relax making the pain less and my fog recede somewhat. My favorite is walking up stairs into an old attic and finding a trunk filled with small boxes. In each box I put a problem in it and lock it away in the trunk until I am feeling ready to deal with it. Then I come back later and take it out and solve the issue. It may sound silly, but it works for me. Another coping tool is movies. I still love to read but when I have trouble concentrating I go to the movies. I get lost in the story and for a couple of hours I am no one but me. (I always take a blanket though because I get cold easily.)

I am no longer working, having taken an early medical retirement about three years ago. I am ambulatory and only on really bad days will I use a cane because my knees tend to go out on me and my hips lock up. I walk a lot slower than I used to and I can't multi-task as well as I once could. I feel like I could probably work some part time job as a secretary or receptionist if something came along. It would give me purpose and a place to be and I could always use the extra money.

I am fortunate that I was able to get my Social Security Disability fairly easily (I had good doctors and kept meticulous records of my own), and I have my retirement but money is always an issue. There is never enough. I was able to keep my medical insurance through the school board and when my SSI came through I got Medicare so my Blue Cross is my supplement. I'm very fortunate in that area. Every month is a game though, who gets paid and who doesn't, or who gets paid in full and who gets a partial payment. And they know me by name at the pay-day advance store! It doesn't help that my husband is sicker now. So that's a daily struggle.

The effects of this disorder on friendships in my life were not so apparent until recently. I went on a weekend trip with a high school friend a few weekends ago and we had a falling out over something stupid, more of a miscommunication really, but she told me "the enemy was working in me" meaning the devil was in me making me sick. That's why I had the fibro, and she would not hear of any other possibility. There is no explaining to people like that so I nixed her off my friends list once and for all. I am sure there are other people who thought I was faking or lazy or whatever, but nothing overt was ever said; it was more just a pulling away and although it was painful, I have learned to live with it and do not miss the people in my life who did not make an attempt to understand me or to care about me regardless of my health. We raised money for all sorts of charities, when someone got sick at school we took them food and helped them in all sort of ways, but not once did anyone do that for me. And yes, I resented it. It hurt my feelings. I felt less than a member of my team.

I love to swim and read, I'm a Facebook stalker, I'm a movie freak, and I love love love my nieces and nephews who spend a lot of time with me doing arts and crafts. Decoupage is our latest craze and we have done some pretty spectacular things! We are also big TV watchers- with money so tight it's our primary form of entertainment and I still love to read. I also have three dogs that I love a lot; they are my babies. I live in a small town and to my knowledge there are no organized support groups for FMS but I read a lot on the subject and talk to my friends who have the disease, comparing notes and commiserating.

When you have Fibromyalgia, and you tell people it is a disease they treat you differently. But because they can't see it or see physical changes like loss of hair in a chemo patient then it doesn't seem real. It is hard to describe FMS in just a few words so that people can understand its devastating effect on its victims. When you say I have cancer people automatically know it's bad, or I have Parkinson's or MS or whatever. These are highly recognized diseases with billions of dollars of research spent annually to search for a cure or to at least make the lives of the sufferers easier. Not to belittle or demean other diseases, but FMS isn't glamorous. No famous person has come out and claimed that he or she has it. I also think the mental illness component that goes along with FMS (depression/bi-polar) is a stigma that makes the "normals" uncomfortable.

I have a friend that I love dearly who believes you can think your way out of depression; I don't even try anymore to convince her otherwise. I do believe that in every case of FMS depression is a factor and that it has to be treated. Sleep is an elusive creature for us and must be dealt with for the body to heal and feel healthy. I remember when I first started taking Ambien I would wake up feeling refreshed and rejuvenated as if I had never been sick at all and I was a new woman! Before Ambien I would wake up feeling like I'd been in a train wreck. I used to have three friends who took turns calling me in the mornings to make sure I was awake and I would still be late to work every single day. Then the Ambien stopped working as well and I was taking two or three at night and suddenly my life revolved around trying to get more. I was addicted and I had to get off them completely. I have finally regained a natural sleep rhythm, although I do get up around three and go back to bed around six- I am making it work.

The only drugs I take now are Klonopin for anxiety which I have a lot of, Paxil for depression and Amitiza for IBS, and the Topomax for FMS. I also take supplements and I firmly believe that is what keeps me going. I take B12 complex, a multivitamin, vitamin D, iron, calcium and protein powder shakes.

I'm not a doctor, but I am a victim of this disease and until more research is done, until more attention is brought to the forefront so that the public is educated we, its victims will continue to suffer in silence and be ridiculed and shuffled aside for promotions we deserve, invitations to gatherings and many, many other things "normals" enjoy.

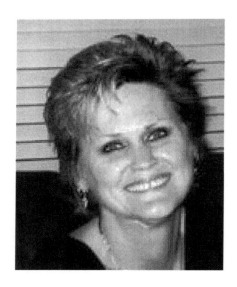

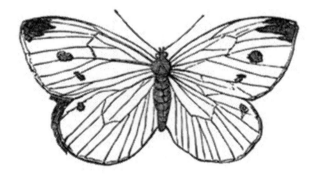

The Girl Inside

By Kelli Glover

Where is that girl inside of me?

That colorful girl I used to be

The bohemian artist so full of life,

 Who could sing and write the day away

Where is that vigor and unstoppable spirit?

The dreams I had so full of promise

I was going to run wild and free

The world was mine, I had so much time

Where are the days when there was not pain

When energy was pouring out of me

I had so much to do

I was going to sing and act

I was going to travel

I was going to write and create beautiful things

And read every book I could handle

They are all distant memories of a time long ago

Before pain and muddled thoughts were my reality

I remember a time when I was respected

Not a woman to be rejected

By an illness people do not believe is real

To be mocked and made fun of by those who you love

The stigma is cruel, if they only knew

The hours you weep in the long, lonely night

While you sit so still, not a sound you ignite

Where are my dreams, they have turned so cold

I don't even hope, I don't know how to anymore

I just try to make it through day by day

Hour by hour

Minute by minute

Hoping each moment may bring, less pain

Less ridicule

Compassion

Love that has been lost to a horrible lot

Pain please go away just for a day

I want to have quality of some sort

Dear God, I pray, are you listening?

I sometimes wonder

Instead of judgment, could you give me a hug

Instead of a lecture, an "I love you"

A gift without a catch

For I never get a break

It would be a kind thing to do

It would make my day and though the pain would not go away

It would ease some stress, nonetheless

Because inside, I am the girl I used to be

For she has never gone away, she is safely tucked away

Perhaps a miracle, perhaps a cure

Perhaps someday, perhaps someday

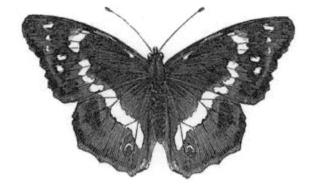

Focus on "CAN!"

By Shelly Bolton

My name is Shelly and I am a 39 year old writer living in north central Texas. My adventure with fibromyalgia began in my mid-twenties, before which I was a fairly healthy person.

My childhood was not an easy one, with bullying as a large part of my early school years. Between bullying and other abuse as a young child, and my parents' divorce during my pre-teens, by the time I reached high school I had my share of emotional scars. I was so blessed, however, to have parents who were very loving. Obviously they were not perfect, but they always made sure I knew they loved me.

As an adult I married a man with whom I had been friends since high school, and the marriage was not good. He was not directly abusive, but was emotionally detached and quite passive-aggressive in his behaviors toward me. My son was born about a year into this marriage, and within the first year after his birth I began having serious health issues, beginning with IBS that was so severe that at times it came close to being life-threatening due to dehydration and similar complications. When my son was three, my husband decided he was done with the marriage and wanted to pursue an alternative lifestyle. We separated pretty much immediately and within a few months he moved to Canada. He has since not been involved in our lives. I often wonder if the stress surrounding the marriage problems was a part of what brought on the initial onset of IBS symptoms.

As time went on I got to the point where I had constant pain, especially in my back. I had experienced some back pain beginning during childhood, due to minor injuries, but it had always resolved in a relatively short period of time. This pain, however, was unrelenting. I spoke with my family doctor about it, and she had the usual tests done; x-ray, CAT scan, MRI; but none showed any serious problems. She prescribed pain meds, anti-inflammatories, and even steroids at one point, but none were particularly helpful. I eventually stopped bothering with trying to find out what it was and decided I was just going to have to live with it- the pain was constant, but at this point was still relatively low-intensity compared with what was to come.

After my divorce I went back to school to work on my bachelor's degree. I was in school full time and working near full time, and was a single mom to a young child, so I did not sleep much during the school terms. I had other symptoms that were beginning to pile up, but I did not really think of them as symptoms. It was just how things were. I also had begun having occasional kidney stones, which are not part of the fibromyalgia constellation of issues, but because they were severe enough at times to be a challenge to my health I think they may have contributed to the progression of the fibro. At one point I was hospitalized for about two weeks and released, then re-hospitalized in a different hospital before attention was given to a stone that was stuck in the ureter, causing it and the kidney to inflame and swell to nearly twice the normal size. After that there was bleeding in the left kidney- due to the stint that was inserted and the damage that had been done- for over a month. I still have problems with pain in the left kidney at times. Since then I have begun taking an herbal supplement called "Stone Free," and drinking about a gallon of water or more each day, and though I still get kidney stones they have remained manageable for the last few years.

During my time back in college I met my current husband, who was also going back to school. We dated for a few years and married, and throughout all of the health issues and everything he has been very supportive and loving. He shows attributes that it never even occurred to me to look for. I like to say that he is "everything I never knew I always wanted." He is not perfect, nor am I, but we have a very loving and happy marriage, and I know that he is a gift from God.

During my hospitalization for the stuck stone I met a nurse who had noticed the variety of symptoms I was experiencing, aside from the pain from the stone. She spoke with me about the possibility of fibromyalgia, explaining what it was and suggesting I see a rheumatologist to have it checked out. I began learning more about it and was very surprised at how closely the list of signs and symptoms fit to my own experiences. There were several things on the list that I had not even paid any attention to up to that point, just thinking they were part of life. It was still a few years before I actually had a doctor that acknowledged fibro as the culprit. Since then I have had a hysterectomy due to a variety of problems, hoping to get significant relief from some of these symptoms. I did get some relief from the immediate monthly issues, but it was not the level of improvement I had hoped for.

Less than a year after my hysterectomy, I got a phone call late in the evening letting me know that my father was being taken by Care-Flight to a hospital in Dallas with a dissecting aortic aneurysm. I was informed that this was extremely critical and immediately made the drive to the hospital, where I waited with my mother, my sister, and my best friend (who is really more of a sister) while my dad underwent a nine-plus-hour surgery overnight. He survived, which is in and of itself a miracle, but had many severe complications which kept him in the ICU in a drug-induced coma for almost a month, and I stayed with him as much as the nurses would allow. That was a stressful time, but miraculously my health seemed to hold up, and I do not regret spending the time being there for my dad when he needed me. Since then, the pain and other issues have seemed to progress and I have developed new symptoms as well. I currently rely primarily on nutrition and herbal supplements to deal with the pain and other issues.

Well I like to think of myself as a positive person. I am a person of strong faith and I look to God for my strength in all of the trial and turmoil. I did not feel that the purpose of my life was to be stuck in bed or on the sofa, just trying to get through each day and the pain that came with it. I had found in all of my research of fibro that though there was information out there, much of it was quite technical in nature, and there was no central resource that just spelled out all of the basics for those of us without a medical degree. I also saw the need for a resource that would put the experience into terms that those who do NOT have the disorder could relate to, since a big issue for many fibromites seems to be that people in their lives just don't get how extreme the effects of this disorder can be. So I figured I wanted to do something positive with what I was going through. I started compiling information from several resources and putting that together with comprehensive descriptions of what the pains and other sensations felt like, as well as throwing in some of my own personal experiences and those of a few other fibro patients. By the time I had finished, I had a book! It was published in February of 2013, and in fact the fibro stories included in it brought such a response from the readers that it is what inspired this very book as well. I like knowing that something positive has come from my difficulties.

One of the main things I have learned in my adult life, and hope to share with others, is that dealing with chronic illness does not have to keep you in a dark and desperate place. My faith has been a cornerstone of strength during some of the most difficult times, and I would encourage anyone looking for that kind of help to seek comfort in God. Also, one of the best ways to keep from drowning in your own problems is to find some way to help someone else. It may be that you aren't physically capable of much, but if you look for it there will be some way that you can serve others around you. Start by looking at what you CAN do. Even if you cannot get out of bed, you can be an encouraging voice to a friend who is going through a hard time. You can go online and offer support and understanding to others who are suffering. I even like to go on Yahoo Answers or similar sites and look under "homework help" for kids who have homework questions I can help with. If you care to find it, there will be something you can offer to help someone.

Another way we can each help each other is to look for ways to raise awareness about this disorder. We need to work together to try and inform the public about fibromyalgia. That is going to be the best way by which we can push toward a goal of getting research dollars into the hands of organizations that are motivated to find a cure. Much of the research up to this point has been done by drug companies whose primary motivation is toward selling us a lifelong treatment. Let's create a surge toward finding other remedies, and get behind the fibromyalgia research organizations that are looking for something other than a pharmaceutical customer.

Write Your Own Fibro Story

_____
_____
_____
_____
_____
_____
_____
_____
_____
_____
_____
_____
_____
_____
_____
_____
_____
_____
_____
_____
_____
_____
_____
_____
_____
_____
_____
_____
_____

Acknowledgements

Thank you so much for reading this book and joining a few fibromites on their journeys in dealing with this condition. We hope that it has encouraged and enlightened you, and maybe even brought a smile to your face at times. To help in raising awareness, please visit http://www.fibromodem.com, and to get information on contributing to fibro research go to http://afsafund.org/ or http://www.nfra.net. You can also feel great that you have already contributed by purchasing this book!

Thanks are also in order to all of the brave fibro fighters who contributed their stories for this project, as well as to those who have helped pull together the finished collection.

To contact Shelly Bolton, please send emails to fibromyalgiajourney@gmail.com.

37981196R00094

Printed in Poland
by Amazon Fulfillment
Poland Sp. z o.o., Wrocław